BEYOND
FEEL
GREAT

BEYOND
FEEL GREAT

THE REAL SYSTEM TO UNLOCK
THE SECRETS TO BETTER HEALTH

DOUG COLLINS

Published: May 2023

Cataloguing in Publication is on file with the Library and Archives Canada

Paperback ISBN: 978-1-7772952-4-0

eBook ISBN: 978-1-7772952-5-7

www.beyondfeelgreat.com

Table of Contents

Preface

I am no stranger to the struggle of feeling great. Throughout my late 20s and 30s, I experienced significant weight fluctuations and increasing chronic health issues like knee and sciatic back pain. Although I believed that I was eating the right way and taking supplements consistently, I received little support for managing my weight gain during those years.

By my early 40s, this was a busy time in my life - I was a corporate executive with a successful 22-year career and a busy young family, raising three children. However, in 2004, I found myself as a single dad with full custody, now responsible for raising these three young children while juggling a corporate job that had me traveling across North America one to two weeks every month. With so much going on in life, my health became the least of my priorities.

In 2008, I received a call from an acquaintance who wanted to share information about a health product. During that period, I found myself struggling with my weight as a single dad raising young children while also managing corporate responsibilities. The demands of both roles had taken a toll on my physical health. I was 100 pounds overweight, and being in my 40s, my unhealthy lifestyle was catching up with me. My knees hurt, my back ached, my blood sugar levels were out of control, and I had a serious cholesterol issue.

What truly motivated me to take my health seriously were the mornings I spent looking in the mirror, seeing a stranger I didn't recognize or like. The fear of growing older and running out of time, just like my parents did, kept haunting me.

On the recommendation of this acquaintance, I decided to try this *fiber matrix drink* they suggested. Within a few months, some of the weight started to come off, and consequently, my chronic pain issues disappeared. People around me began to notice the changes in my appearance and started inquiring about what I had been doing. Feeling much better and knowing that I was finally on the right path brought me immense relief.

As a result of a corporate merger and downsizing in 2010, I made the decision to leave my career and pursue my long-held dream of becoming self-employed, working from home. That decision marked the beginning of my journey here, where my focus has since been on learning and applying the health principles found in this book, *Beyond Feel Great*, in my own life; and to actively be sharing this message as an option for others.

Second Chance for a New Beginning

In 2015, while attending a health conference, I had a life-transformative experience. At that conference, I met men who were a decade older than me but in much better health, which made me reflect on my own health journey to date, the results I had achieved, and the fact that I hadn't inherited good health genetics, which was part of the underlying cause of some of my health struggles.

My dad had passed away at the age of 66 from prostate cancer, and when he was 57, he had a massive heart attack, with eighty percent of his arteries clogged. My mom had passed away at 69 from heart disease after spending the last decade of her life with chronic sickness. I had also lost an older sister in her 40s to childhood brain cancer, and by the time I was 10 years old, all my grandparents had already passed away.

As I was inspired by the health transformation results I saw at the conference, I realized that, while I had experienced great results up to that point in time, I had still settled for average health. These guys had what I wanted, and I wasn't willing to settle for anything less.

It was at that moment during the conference I made a decision: I was going to do everything possible to break the patterns from my last couple of generations and maintain optimal health as I entered my 50s, 60s, and beyond. That is when I knew I needed more support.

I enlisted the help of a transformation coach who guided and motivated me on my journey toward my new health goals. They taught me how to make simple, lasting changes to the way I eat, exercise, and live my life. As a result, I developed healthier habits and routines over the next two years, leading to the best health I've ever had.

During this time, I lost 100 pounds (45 kg) and gained 20 pounds (9 kg) of lean muscle. Having a coach helped me to stay focused, get past my mental blocks, and the experience taught me how to stack healthy habits that will now serve me for a lifetime.

Soon after this period, I visited my doctor for a check-up. To my amazement, he said to me, "I've never seen a patient lose 100 pounds and improve their blood lipids so much." He also told me that my risk of developing heart disease had dropped to less than 5%, and my diabetes risk was now 0%. Right then, I felt a strong sense of pride and achievement, which confirmed that prioritizing my health and well-being was the right decision.

Coping with Life Crisis

In late 2017, my life took an unexpected turn when my wife's sister was diagnosed with grade IV glioblastoma, a fast-growing and aggressive brain tumor. She moved in with us following emergency surgery, and as the self-employed head of the family who worked from home, I took on the responsibility of coordinating all front-line healthcare communication, doctors' appointments, and treatments.

I also became her primary driver, chauffeuring her to medical appointments and treatment sessions. This role consumed my life for the next thirteen months, as I supported my sister-in-law and tried to maintain balance in my own life.

Much like the life-changing experience years ago when I became a single dad raising three young children, the focus on myself became my last priority. During that year-long period, I was constantly consumed with my sister-in-law's medical needs, and my own health suffered as a result.

I struggled to find time or motivation to engage in physical activity or eat well, causing both my health and home business to spiral downward and placing significant strain on my marriage to my wonderful wife, as my wife and I struggled to balance caring for her sister with our own needs and priorities. At times, it felt like everything was spiraling out of control.

Perhaps you're reading this and can relate: we all face life challenges. Yes, I get it – life struggles are real, and they will get in the way! I understand that life challenges can cause setbacks, and I too experienced some setbacks during that year. I gained just a few pounds back, but thankfully, the healthier habits I had developed helped me avoid returning to my former unhealthy self.

Navigating Transitions: Overcoming Pandemic Obstacles

By late 2019, life began to settle back into somewhat of a routine. By then, three children had grown up and moved away. It was at that time when we felt a pull for a significant lifestyle change that included relocation back to my hometown. In November of that year, we put the house up for sale, believing that if it was meant to happen, the house would sell quickly. The house sold in just a few days, and we embarked on a new chapter in life, full of goals, dreams, and the excitement of a healthy lifestyle in my hometown.

However, little did I know that this transition would bring more unexpected challenges, just like it did for everyone in the world.

In March 2020, the pandemic lockdown had a profound impact on my business focus, mobility, and enjoyment of playing sports like hockey and squash. Despite these challenges, I took advantage of my time indoors to focus on writing and publishing my first book. The result was my first published book that became an Amazon bestseller in August 2020.

While writing and publishing a bestseller was a great achievement, it took a toll on my physical health. Due to the lockdown restrictions, I was sitting for long hours, which led to a more sedentary lifestyle than I was accustomed to. As the pandemic continued, I also noticed the adverse effects it had on the well-being of others, which prompted me to realize the importance of not just physical health, but also mental and emotional well-being in creating a balanced, fulfilling life.

This realization inspired me to shift my focus and become an early adopter and innovator in a health and wellness movement that emphasizes achieving and sustaining optimal health through a combination of two food-based products and a time-restricted eating schedule.

I realized that achieving a balanced and fulfilling life required not just physical health, but also mental and emotional well-being. It was clear that I needed to take charge and make another significant change in my life. So, in late 2020, I decided to shift my focus from publishing to prioritizing my own health and well-being, while also actively sharing with others how to feel great despite the challenges presented by the pandemic.

My new mission inspired me to become an early adopter and innovator in a health and wellness movement that focuses on achieving and sustaining optimal health through a combination of two food-based products and a time-restricted eating schedule. Through my own experiences, I learned the value of having the right tools, support system, roadmap, and accountability to guide and motivate us on our journey towards well-being. I am now passionate about sharing these insights with others and helping them achieve their health goals.

Beyond Feel Great is an extension of this health and wellness movement as my personal experiences have led me to appreciate the importance of having the right tools, support system, roadmap, and accountability to guide and motivate us on our journey towards well-being.

In this book, I share my story, insights, and strategies with you, in the hopes of empowering you to transform your life. My hope is for this book to inspire you to break free from unhealthy patterns and take control of your health, just as I did.

Every individual's journey is unique, and I understand that there will be setbacks and challenges along the way. However, by sharing the experiences and the insights I've gained, I hope to provide support, encouragement, and motivation. Together, we can navigate the winding path called Life to find better health and happiness, and ultimately, create lasting, positive change in our lives.

Introduction

Welcome to *Beyond Feel Great*, a book that provides a unique perspective on achieving optimal health. Unlike the abundance of other health-related books, coaching programs, and supplement marketers out there, the message and information in this book offer clear insights and evidence-based principles for overcoming health challenges and achieving your health goals.

In *Beyond Feel Great*, we'll lay the groundwork for long-term health by focusing on three fundamental elements of a healthy lifestyle: proper nutrition, regular exercise, and mindful lifestyle choices. Instead of chasing after fad diets or so-called "miracle" supplements, we'll explore sustainable approaches to achieving optimal health.

We'll delve into the link between glucose and insulin levels in the body, a connection that can contribute to chronic health issues. This section will also cover the impact of carbohydrates on blood sugar levels and the effects of processed foods on our overall well-being.

Insulin resistance is becoming increasingly common. We'll examine its impact on our bodies and discuss strategies to prevent it. Additionally, we'll look at the relationship between the hormone insulin and weight management, and explore the connection between insulin and blood pressure.

Metabolic flexibility, or the body's ability to switch between different energy sources, is a key aspect of health. We'll explore ways to improve this flexibility, including the benefits of intermittent fasting on overall well-being.

Essential nutrients are vital for optimal health, and we'll explore the keys to obtaining them through diet. We'll also examine the benefits of an active lifestyle and provide practical tips on how to incorporate movement into your daily routine.

We'll discuss healthy habits and practices that promote long-term health and success, and highlight common mistakes people make when trying to improve their health. More importantly, we'll provide guidance on how to avoid these pitfalls.

Finally, *Beyond Feel Great* provides actionable steps you can take to start your health journey and achieve lasting success. This book is more than a guide; it's a companion on your path to a healthier life.

I invite you to engage with this book, read each section carefully, and take action on the principles discussed. By doing so, you'll gain the knowledge and tools needed to transform your health and achieve your goals. Let's begin this journey towards better health together. Welcome to *Beyond Feel Great*!

Chapter 1

Beyond Fad Diets and Quick-Fixes

Today's fast-paced, high-stress, post-pandemic society has taken a toll on our well-being, with the prevalence of processed and fast foods, sedentary jobs, and easy access to technology. As a result, these factors have contributed to the growing incidence of chronic health issues such as obesity, diabetes, high blood pressure, and high cholesterol.

Never before in history has it been so crucial to prioritize our health and find a balance amid the many challenges of modern living. Sedentary lifestyles and unhealthy diets are contributing to the escalating obesity and diabetes crises, leading individuals to gain weight and develop chronic conditions at increasingly younger ages.[1]

With our hectic lifestyles today, many people seek quick results, especially, when it comes to weight loss, controlling blood sugars in situations of type 2 diabetes, and feeling great for overall health.[2] However, when it comes to improving our health and losing weight, society is often lured into quick fixes and fad diet plans to help achieve these goals.

This often results in only short-term results, if any, at all. It's important to understand that each individual's body responds differently and at its own pace, so immediate changes may not necessarily yield rapid outcomes in achieving health goals. Instead, it is always wise to focus on implementing changes in a healthy and sustainable manner, with an emphasis on balance and moderation.

Throughout this book, we will explore the following topics to help you prioritize your health:

- The impact of sedentary lifestyles and unhealthy diets on our health.

- The growing prevalence of chronic health issues like obesity and diabetes.

- The importance of sustainable, balanced changes for long-term health.

- Tips and practices for gently guiding the body towards positive changes.

Ultimately, regardless of our busy schedules, circumstances, cultural differences, or geographic location, our bodies operate in much the same way and require us to follow the same basic science-based principles for optimal health. By the end of this book, you will have a deeper understanding of how to prioritize your health in a sustainable and effective way and how to apply these principles to your own unique situation.

The Dual Crisis: Obesity and Diabetes

We currently face a dual crisis of obesity and diabetes. According to recent data from the CDC, the prevalence of obesity in Americans rose from 30.5% in 1999-2000 to 42.4% in 2017-2018, emphasizing the gravity of the situation.[3]

Researchers at Tufts University have uncovered a critical health crisis that necessitates urgent action. Only 7% of the

U.S. adult population maintains good cardiometabolic health.[4] Cardiometabolic health involves various risk factors, such as type 2 diabetes and insulin resistance, cardiovascular disease, cholesterol levels, high blood pressure, as well as issues related to overweight and obesity.

In order to be classified as having 'good cardiometabolic health,' an individual must exhibit optimal levels across all five components, encompassing body fat tissue (adiposity), blood glucose, blood lipids, blood pressure, and clinical cardiovascular disease. Alarmingly, 93% of U.S. adults do not meet these criteria as having good cardiometabolic health.[5]

The pandemic has further exacerbated these concerning statistics, with 42% of U.S. adults who participated in the American Psychological Association's 2021 Stress in America Poll, responded with unintended weight gain since the pandemic's onset. Among this group, the average weight gain was 29 pounds, while 10% indicated they had gained over 50 pounds during this challenging period.[6]

The CDC also announced on September 15, 2021, that the number of states with high obesity prevalence, defined as at least 35% of residents with obesity, has nearly doubled since 2018.[7]

According to the International Diabetes Federation, diabetes around the world is 'spiraling out of control' with 1 in 10 adults living with diabetes globally in 2021.[8] The IDF website reports that the more we know, the worse the picture is, with diabetes being a global killer and one of the leading causes of premature death.[9]

Diabetes is a significant global challenge to the health and well-being of individuals, families, and societies. Diabetes claims lives and causes disability, with 6.7 million deaths in 2021, 1 person dies of diabetes every 5 seconds.[10] People with prediabetes may develop type 2 diabetes within three years if they do not take steps to prevent it.[11]

According to the Center for Disease Control, individuals have a higher probability of developing prediabetes and type 2 diabetes if they have certain risk factors. These risk factors include being 45 years of age or older, being overweight, having a family history of type 2 diabetes, engaging in physical activity fewer than three times per week, or having a history of gestational diabetes during pregnancy or giving birth to a baby weighing more than 9 pounds.[12]

From Social Media Hype to Quick-Fix Supplements

I created this book because I have observed many people trying various dietary and supplement routines they discovered through social media, but not achieving their desired results within a few months. This frustration often leads them to give up and switch to something else. However, unlocking the secrets to better health requires balance and consistency to create a sustainable healthy lifestyle.

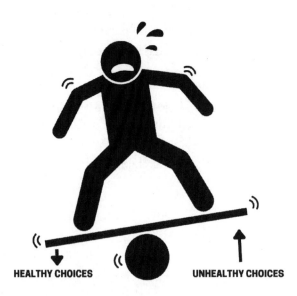

HEALTHY CHOICES   UNHEALTHY CHOICES

Too often, we look for a quick fix or a fad diet without taking the time to focus on the basics of health. I understand this tendency and interest, because I've been there myself. However, based on my personal experience and research, this approach doesn't align with a focus for long term health. That's why we need to shift our mindset.

Unfortunately, in today's world, the influence of social media and online marketeers have contributed to the circulation of misleading information and profiteering on people's desire (and struggle) for health. Often, they suggest that consuming certain supplements or eliminating certain foods will enable us to eat as we please while still resolving weight and chronic health issues.

It's alluring to believe that we can indulge in whatever we please without consequence and that just taking "supplements" will suffice, neglecting the need for any dietary or lifestyle adjustments. This marketing strategy often serves one purpose: to generate more sales of whatever is being sold!

In my experience and extensive research, nutrition products can be used as a foundation to support any health journey. While supplements can be tools for enhancing results, they should not be viewed as a single replacement in creating a healthy and balanced lifestyle. The message found in this book, *Beyond Feel Great*, will address the importance of a balanced diet, regular exercise, stress management, and other lifestyle factors that are essential for sustained success.

As you read this book, you will see that I make reference to science-based nutrition products that have been a foundation to support my health journey. However, it's important to note that as good as these products are, they alone are not a magic solution.

To achieve optimal health and well-being, we must make an active intention to take responsibility for all aspects of our lifestyle and create balance. As good as any products may be, as valuable tools for enhancing results, they should not be viewed as the sole tool for creating a healthy and balanced lifestyle, which is essential for sustained success. Just like the saying "we can't out-exercise a bad diet," the same goes for supplements: "we can't out-supplement a bad diet."

In this book, we will take more of a holistic approach to health that I have personally learned and followed, and thousands of others are following to achieve lasting results. As well, whenever I make reference to the products I personally use and recommend, you will notice I have omitted the product and company names. This was not an attempt to withhold information, but rather a measure to maintain objectivity, avoid potential legal or compliance issues with company policies and government regulators.

"I strongly believe in the products I personally use and recommend. It's important to emphasize that nutrition supplements are just one part of a comprehensive approach to health and wellness. That's why throughout this book, it will emphasize the importance of a balanced diet, regular exercise, stress management, and other lifestyle factors that are essential for sustained success.

The Foundation of Optimal Health

The purpose of this book is to emphasize our accountability for the decisions we make regarding the food we eat, the way we think, and the physical activity we engage in. This understanding forms the basis of the title of this book, *Beyond Feel Great*. Throughout these pages, we will explore what is required for achieving optimal health and making lasting changes that enhance our health and well-being.

The health priorities pyramid below illustrates the importance of taking a bottom-up approach to health and wellness. To achieve optimal health, we need to build a strong foundation that emphasizes understanding our lifestyle habits, dietary behaviors, and consistency, and by doing so, we can make meaningful and lasting changes that lead to optimal health and well-being.

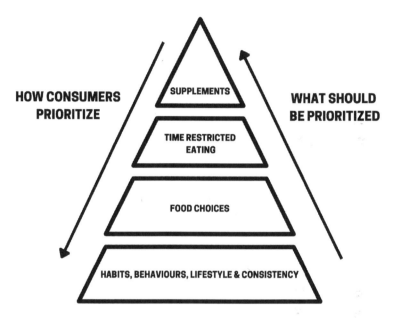

By establishing a strong foundation, we can use other aspects of the pyramid, such as food choices, time-restricted eating, and science-based supplements, to improve our health and achieve long-term results. Our daily food choices play a crucial role in our health and well-being, and the overconsumption of ultra-processed foods is often the root cause of chronic health issues.

This book will guide you towards making lasting changes to improve your health. Let's explore the role of diet and lifestyle in our health journey together, starting with the next chapter's focus on consistently high glucose and insulin levels. Join me on this journey towards better health!

Chapter 2

Glucose-Insulin: The Vicious Cycle

You might be wondering why I'm starting with the subject of glucose. Perhaps you're thinking that this only applies to those who are diabetic. However, this couldn't be further from the truth. Understanding how chronic conditions begin, starts with the basics of how our bodies process the food we eat. It all starts with the foods we eat and digest, and how we unknowingly continue this cycle over a long period of time.

When we eat, our food is broken down into glucose, which then enters our bloodstream. Our bodies require glucose and fat as sources of energy, and glucose is absorbed into the body through digestion.

The hormone insulin, produced by the pancreas, helps regulate our blood sugar levels by moving glucose from our blood into our cells for energy. After consuming carbohydrate-rich foods, the beta cells in the pancreas produce insulin to control blood glucose levels. Insulin signals our fat and muscle cells to absorb glucose from the bloodstream, reducing high blood glucose levels. However, when we overeat and consume more glucose than our body needs, the excess glucose is stored in fat cells, leading to weight gain.

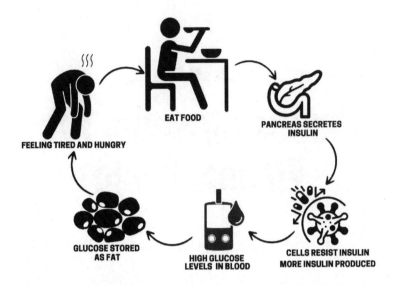

EAT FOOD

PANCREAS SECRETES INSULIN

FEELING TIRED AND HUNGRY

GLUCOSE STORED AS FAT

HIGH GLUCOSE LEVELS IN BLOOD

CELLS RESIST INSULIN MORE INSULIN PRODUCED

Now, here's the tricky part: insulin leaves our bodies at a much slower rate than glucose, and our bodies cannot access fat stores when insulin is present in our bloodstream. If we consume a high-carbohydrate meal, we may feel hungry and irritable before the insulin has left our bloodstream, causing us to eat again and release more insulin.

This cycle can persist throughout the day, constantly exposing our bodies to insulin, which can have a detrimental effect. It not only prevents weight loss but also causes us to age faster and increases insulin resistance. By understanding how glucose and the hormone insulin work together, we can begin to see how they are connected to many chronic health problems like pre-diabetes, type 2 diabetes, high blood pressure, and high cholesterol.[13]

After our cells have used up the glucose, there is still insulin left circulating in the blood. This extra insulin makes our blood sugar go too low, which makes us feel hungry again, starting the glucose and insulin cycle all over. This condition is known as hypoglycemia. Hypoglycemia is most often recognized in diabetic patients who take glucose or insulin medication. However, it can occur in almost anyone. Perhaps from time to time, you have experienced these symptoms of hypoglycemia like extreme hunger (hangry), dizziness, confusion, headaches or brain fog, nausea, sweatiness or shakiness.

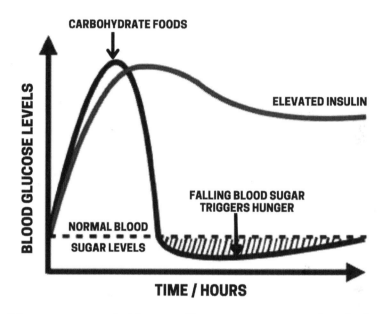

Then, we eat to feel better. Glucose increases, and with that, a corresponding increase in insulin. We feel better for a short time, and the cycle begins again. Over years and decades of this continuous cycle, unknowingly, our body loses its natural balance of glucose and insulin, resulting in a situation called insulin resistance. This is when we start developing chronic health issues, such as weight gain and prediabetes. Despite all our efforts to lose weight, the glucose-insulin connection makes it almost impossible for our bodies to burn body fat for energy, making it extremely challenging to lose weight permanently.

By understanding this little-known condition called insulin resistance, and its correlation and risks to many chronic conditions, we can make smarter choices about our health and take action to prevent and manage health problems. In this book, we'll discuss the changes we can make in our diets, such as eating more fiber, and how being more active can help us fight these health issues.

Prediabetes: The Alarming Reality

Back in the 1920s, two-thirds of the world's population was malnourished. But now, things have changed, and only one-fourth of the world's population don't get enough to eat.[14] Unfortunately, the foods we eat today, particularly processed foods, can be just as harmful to our health as not eating enough. These foods cause our blood sugar levels to rise quickly, which is detrimental to our well-being.[15]

The Center for Disease Control (CDC) reports that over 1 in 3 people worldwide have prediabetes, with more than 84% of those individuals unaware that they have it. Shockingly, almost 50% of people diagnosed with prediabetes go on to develop diabetes.[16]

	A1C	FASTING GLUCOSE		2 HRS POST MEAL	
		mg/dl	mmol/l	mg/dl	mmol/l
DIABETES	6.5 & ABOVE	≥126	≥7	≥200	≥11.1
PRE DIABETES	5.7 to 6.4	100 to 126	5.6 to 7	140 to 199	7.77 to 11
HEALTHY	BELOW 5.6	≤126	3.89 to 5.5	≤139	≤7.72

Prediabetes is a prevalent condition affecting millions of people worldwide. It is a chronic condition that links to lifestyle habits such as a sedentary lifestyle and a diet high in processed foods and added sugars. If left untreated or poorly managed, type 2 diabetes can cause several long-term health complications.[17]

It's crucial to recognize the alarming reality of prediabetes and take steps to prevent or manage the condition before it progresses into type 2 diabetes. As we begin to understand how we digest and utilize glucose from the foods we eat, we are realizing that it has a dramatic impact on our long-term health and the management of chronic conditions. By adopting a healthier lifestyle, we can avoid the long-term complications that come with developing diabetes if left unaddressed.[18]

Type 2 Diabetes: The Global Impact

As we are beginning to understand, the development of type 2 diabetes and its complications does not occur in isolation. There is a strong connection between insulin resistance, type 2 diabetes, and other chronic conditions and health problems, such as obesity, hypertension, and high cholesterol levels. These disorders often share common risk factors, such as poor diet and lack of physical activity, creating a vicious cycle that further impairs the body's ability to regulate blood sugar levels and maintain overall health. This can increase the risk of developing even more complications, such as heart disease and nerve damage.[19]

As we will discuss in detail in a later chapter, how insulin resistance lies at the heart of this issue. For now its important to fully understand that when cells in the muscles, fat, and liver become resistant to insulin, they no longer respond effectively to the hormone's signals to absorb glucose from the bloodstream. As a result, blood glucose levels rise, prompting the pancreas to produce even more insulin in an attempt to compensate for the resistance. Over time, the pancreas becomes overworked and unable to produce sufficient insulin, worsening the problem.[20]

The number of people with type 2 diabetes worldwide has more than doubled over the past three decades.[21] It's become a chronic health condition that affects millions of people worldwide, posing a significant challenge to healthcare system and is having a significant impact on human life.[22] Globally it is projected to increase to 643 million by 2030, representing 7.7% of the total adult population of the world aged 20–79 years.[23]

In the United States, according to the Center for Disease Control (CDC), over 37 million Americans have diabetes (about 1 in 10), and about 90-95% of them have type 2 diabetes.[24] Type 2 diabetes most often develops in people over the age of 45, but it is becoming more common in children, teens, and young adults.[25]

The Role of Glucose Medications

In diabetes treatment, the first-line treatment is to use medications to regulate blood sugar levels. Various forms of medication, such as pills or injections, are available, with the selection tailored to the patient's needs. Metformin is a widely used medication for type 2 diabetes due to its rapid blood sugar-lowering effects. It functions by decreasing glucose production in the liver and enhancing the body's insulin sensitivity.

While some people with type 2 diabetes can initially attain near-normal blood sugar levels through medications, many require multiple medications and even insulin therapy. The choice of medication depends on various factors, including blood sugar levels and any co-existing health conditions.

Dietary and lifestyle changes are often recommended, but the focus is still on treatment using drugs. Even with these drugs being the focus for treatment, it is not a cure, and its long-term effectiveness varies among individuals.

There is no general consensus on the optimal medications, or combinations, for blood sugar management and side effect prevention. To investigate this, a National Institute of Health-funded study compared drugs combinations used alongside metformin. During the five years of the study, all four combinations led to improved blood sugar levels during the early study period, with liraglutide and long-acting insulin being the most effective in maintaining target blood glucose levels.[26]

However, its important to note that the study revealed nearly 75% of participants could not sustain their blood glucose targets, emphasizing the difficulties in diabetes management long term with drugs alone. The study's purpose was to equip healthcare providers with information on long-term management, taking into account glucose control, medication tolerance, and other health considerations.

While dietary intake and lifestyle are significant factors in managing type 2 diabetes, the medical focus is still on managing the disease with drugs. It's worth noting that despite all this focus on diabetes drug treatments, type 2 diabetes kills at least twice as many Americans as opioid overdoses on any given day.[27]

Morning Glucose: After Sleeping all Night

People with type 2 diabetes often check their morning fasting blood glucose levels to help monitor their blood sugar control. This is because overnight, the body's glucose levels can fluctuate significantly, and for people with type 2 diabetes, their bodies may struggle to regulate glucose levels on their own.

Checking blood glucose levels in the morning before eating or drinking anything can provide insight into how well their body is controlling glucose. It can also help them make informed decisions about food choices and medication adjustments throughout the day to maintain blood sugar levels. By regularly monitoring their morning fasting blood glucose levels, and taking into account what was consumed for foods in the previous day, we can have great insight into how the body is working – especially into understanding the level of insulin resistance.

High blood sugar in the morning after a night of sleeping is what is known as the dawn phenomenon, which is the end result of a combination of natural body changes throughout the night. The effects of the dawn phenomenon can vary from person to person, even from day to day. According to the American Diabetes Association, the dawn phenomenon happens between 5:00 a.m. and 8:00 a.m. Some people experience an extended dawn phenomenon, which can last until mid-morning.[28]

The boost in morning blood sugar is the body's way of ensuring that there is enough energy to get up and start the day. For those with higher insulin resistance, such as those with prediabetes or type 2 diabetes, the body may not be able to use its insulin to counteract the increase in morning glucose. This disrupts the delicate balance, and sugar readings can be too high by morning.

High morning blood sugar levels are a result of changes and reactions that happen while the body is sleeping. The body uses glucose as one source of energy, and it is important to have enough extra energy to be able to wake up in the morning. For a period of time in the early morning hours, usually between 3 a.m. and 8 a.m., the body starts churning out stored glucose to prepare for the upcoming day.

Even if your last 24 hours have been very low-carb, high morning glucose levels can still occur because the body needs to use up its stored glucose first. This is called 'metabolic inflexibility', and it is estimated that only 15% of the population is metabolically flexible, meaning their body can easily switch from using glucose to using fat for energy.[29]

Typically, the body undergoes natural hormonal changes in the morning that result in a blood sugar boost, occurring in individuals with or without diabetes. For those without diabetes, the body produces extra insulin to maintain balance, going largely unnoticed. However, for individuals with diabetes, their body's insulin response is different, causing fasting blood sugar levels to rise even when they are consistently taking drugs and following a strict diet. Fortunately, there is room for improvement, like incorporating more fiber into the diet. This single step alone, serves as a valuable clinically-proven strategy for managing blood sugar levels in type 2 diabetes.[30]

Fiber's Role in Glucose Control

Incorporating more fiber into the diet has been proven to be the most effective long-term, studies have shown this strategy alone can have a dramatic impact for managing blood sugar levels in individuals with prediabetes, type 2 diabetes, and for maintaining overall health. Fiber, an indigestible carbohydrate, is found in plant-based foods like fruits, vegetables, whole grains, and legumes. It is classified as either soluble or insoluble.

Soluble fiber, found in foods like oats, barley, and beans, dissolves in water and forms a gel-like substance in the digestive system, slowing sugar absorption in the bloodstream. Insoluble fiber, found in foods like wheat bran, whole wheat, and nuts, doesn't dissolve in water and adds bulk to the stool, promoting regular bowel movements.

Fiber helps manage blood sugar levels by slowing glucose absorption, improving insulin sensitivity, and promoting satiety, which aids weight management. Adults should consume 25-30 grams of fiber daily, with some experts recommending 50 grams or more. According to the USDA, more than 90 percent of adults do not meet the recommended minimum intake of dietary fiber; however, many still fall short of this goal.[31]

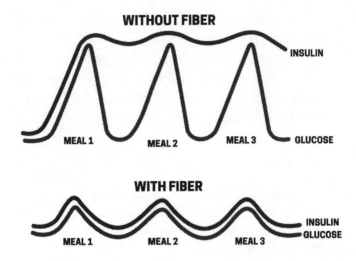

To increase fiber intake, it is important to focus on vegetables, whole grains, legumes, nuts, and seeds. For most people, this can be challenging to consume on a consistent basis, often resulting in an interest in enhancing their health by adding a fiber supplement to their diet. However, it is important to understand the differences in the most popular supplements, as there is a vast difference in formulations, effectiveness, and science-based results. It's not always just about the price and convenience.

One of the most common fiber supplements is a soluble fiber from psyllium husks, which works by stimulating peristalsis like a bulk-forming laxative and slowing intestinal transit. Although fiber supplements with psyllium husks are gentle laxatives, there are mixed reviews on the benefits of taking them long-term and for their effects on blood sugars.[32]

The *fiber matrix drink* that I personally use and recommend is a food supplement designed to be taken with food, as it provides the necessary daily fiber intake and is clinically proven to promote stable blood sugar levels by slowing glucose absorption.[33] It also supports healthy cholesterol levels and digestion while providing essential nutrients for efficient body functioning.[34]

A 2011 study conducted on this *fiber matrix drink* at the University of Sydney in Australia showed that it reduced blood glucose levels by 20% and blood insulin levels by 13%. Two servings reduced blood glucose levels by 28% and blood insulin levels by 27%. In this study, they used white bread, white rice, and instant mashed potatoes as the medium to measure the glucose impact.[35]

In another study from 2002, published in the journal Metabolism and was endorsed by the American Heart Association, concluded that the *fiber matrix drink* was very beneficial for type 2 diabetics and people with high cholesterol in general, who want to reduce cholesterol in a natural way.[36] In that study, fasting blood glucose was reduced by 20.4% and post-meal glucose was reduced 43.7%. The University of Nevada conducted a clinical trial using the *fiber matrix drink*, and they showed it had a beneficial effect on glucose control in insulin-resistant rats.[37] There have been many other studies conducted at Stanford School of Medicine, Columbia University, Cleveland Clinic, Emory University, UCLA, and the University of Utah.

The focus on drugs for long-term management of blood sugar and insulin levels has proven to be unsuccessful. Unfortunately, this has led to a neglect of fiber as a highly effective first-line treatment for conditions like type 2 diabetes. Fiber has been shown to slow down glucose absorption, improve insulin sensitivity, and promote satiety, all of which help prevent overeating and improve blood sugar control. To incorporate more fiber into your diet, try adding fiber-rich foods and consider adding fiber with supplements such as the *fiber matrix drink*. By taking these steps, you can reduce your risk of complications associated with type 2 diabetes and take control of your health. For more information on managing blood sugar with dietary fiber and the *fiber matrix drink*, visit beyondfeelgreatbook.com. Start making positive changes for your health today!

Chapter 3

Glycemic Index: Carbs Made Simple

The old adage, "we are what we eat," rings especially true when it comes to carbohydrates. Not all carbs are the same, and selecting the right ones can greatly influence the glucose-insulin cycle we covered in the previous chapter.

The glycemic index is a system that assigns a numerical value to carbohydrates based on how rapidly they elevate your blood sugar levels. Lower numbers indicate slower digestion and absorption, resulting in a smaller effect on blood sugar. The higher numbers signify quicker digestion and absorption, leading to a more substantial impact on blood sugar.

The Glycemic Index: Its Impact on Health

The glycemic index (GI) was developed by Dr. David Jenkins, a nutrition professor at the University of Toronto, in the early 1980s.[38] Dr. Jenkins and his team introduced the concept of the glycemic index to assist individuals with diabetes in managing their blood sugar levels more effectively by selecting the appropriate types of carbohydrates. Initially, they tested the GI on a small group of volunteers before broadening their research to encompass larger groups of people with diabetes and various other health issues.

Carbohydrates are an essential macronutrient that provides energy to our bodies. However, not all carbohydrates are created equal. Some are quickly digested and absorbed, leading to rapid spikes in blood sugar levels, while others are slowly digested and absorbed, resulting in a more gradual and sustained release of glucose into the bloodstream.

The glycemic index measures how quickly foods are digested and absorbed, and assigns them a score between 0 and 100. Foods with a high GI score (70 or above) cause rapid spikes in blood sugar levels, while low GI foods (55 or below) are digested more slowly and have a more gradual impact on blood sugar levels.

Choosing low GI foods can reduce the glucose-insulin cycle we covered earlier. This can help in keeping glucose and insulin levels lower throughout the day, resulting in better weight control, avoidance of blood sugar spikes and lows that can lead to hypoglycemia, and a reduced risk of developing type 2 diabetes.[39] On the other hand, consuming high GI foods can lead to weight gain, increased appetite, and insulin resistance, ultimately leading to type 2 diabetes and other health problems.

Glycemic Index Research

The glycemic index is well-known and utilized by nutritionists, researchers, and healthcare professionals globally; however, as consumers, we still lack a complete understanding of its significance, particularly in relation to blood sugar control and insulin sensitivity.

The University of Sydney is a public research university located in Sydney, Australia. Founded in 1850 as Australia's first university, it is regarded as one of the world's leading universities.[40] It is also home to the International Glycemic Index (GI) Database maintained by the Human Nutrition Unit, and the Sydney University Glycemic Index Research Service (SUGiRS).[41]

The Sydney University Glycemic Index Research Service (SUGiRS) has an established commercial GI testing laboratory, where they test foods for their glycemic index, insulin index, satiety response, and other metabolic parameters.

The glycemic index is based on the rate at which carbohydrates are digested and absorbed, and how quickly they raise blood sugar levels. This rate is influenced by a variety of factors, including the type of carbohydrate, the fiber content, the level of processing, and the presence of fat and protein in the meal.

Low GI foods, such as whole grains, fruits, and vegetables, are high in fiber and take longer to digest, resulting in a slower and more sustained release of glucose into the bloodstream. High GI foods, such as white bread, sugary drinks, and processed snacks, are low in fiber and are quickly digested and absorbed, leading to rapid spikes in blood sugar levels.

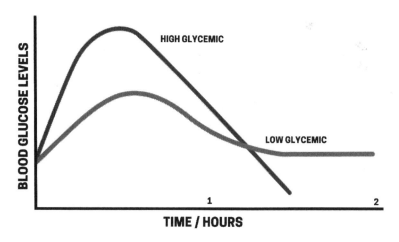

The glycemic index can be a useful tool for managing blood sugar levels, especially for people concerned about prediabetes and type 2 diabetes. By choosing low GI foods, we can maintain better control over our blood sugar levels and reduce our risk of complications.[42]

Glycemic Index: Making Better Choices

Using the glycemic index to make better food choices can be relatively straightforward. The key is to choose low GI foods, and avoid high GI foods as much as possible. Some examples of low GI foods include: legumes (e.g., lentils, chickpeas, black beans). Some examples of high GI foods to limit or avoid include: potatoes, breads, pastries and often packaged ultra-processed foods.

It is important to note that the glycemic index is just one factor to consider when making food choices. Some foods that may seem healthy can still be high glycemic and in some instances not be as beneficial for individuals because of the glucose response. For example, although watermelon, banana, and blueberries are considered healthy, they all have a similar GI rating to white pasta noodles, which are known to be high glycemic.

The glycemic index of the foods we eat can be influenced by other factors, such as the presence of foods with fiber, protein, and healthy fats. The presence of these essential macronutrients in the meal can slow down the absorption of glucose and reduce its impact on blood sugar levels, even in higher GI foods.[43]

The glycemic index is a powerful tool that can help you make better food choices and improve our health. However in today's fast-paced ultra-processed world, it can be challenging to consistently make low glycemic food choices for every single meal.

In fact, studies have shown that eating low glycemic foods with more fiber are digested slower than carbs that do not contain adequate fiber. Considering most of us require 25 to 30 grams of fiber a day, it is difficult to achieve through a low glycemic health dietary intake alone. That's why the *fiber matrix drink* that I use and reference in the book, as a premeal drink, has been clinically-proven to make a difference in managing blood glucose.[44]

Ensuring we get enough of the right kind of fiber with our meals is important because it slows down how fast glucose gets absorbed in our bodies, helps our bodies use insulin better, and makes us feel full so we don't overeat.[45] In addition, as mentioned, studies have shown that this *fiber matrix drink* is very beneficial as a pre-meal drink in lowering the glycemic index of the foods we eat, making it a great way for those who want to control their glycemic impact of the foods we eat.

By choosing low GI foods, avoiding high GI foods, and supplementing with the *fiber matrix drink* as a premeal fiber drink, we can better control our blood glucose levels, feel fuller, and move towards our health goals more quickly without living with an unsustainable dietary lifestyle.

The glycemic index can be a useful guide to help make more conscientious decisions about which foods to include in our meals. To help you incorporate the glycemic index into your daily routine, you can download a handy *Food Guide* that breaks down all foods into three categories: Foods to Avoid (high GI), Foods in Moderation (medium GI), and Foods to Enjoy (low GI). Take an important step towards better health and download the *Food Guide* at beyondfeelgreatbook.com.

Chapter 4

_e e_

Ultra-Processed Foods: Pleasure vs Health

Before we go any further, it is time to address the elephant in the room - our present-day food landscape! If we look back over the last couple of generations, the food we eat has undergone a considerable transformation from wholesome, nutrient-dense foods to ultra-processed, easily accessible options. Consequently, much of the dietary intake has moved towards more refined sugars, harmful fats, and excessive amounts of sodium. Our lifestyles today, combined with the prevalence and ease of fast food, make it increasingly easy to opt for unhealthy meals on the go, leading to a significant increase in chronic health issues.[46]

Processed Foods: The Dangers

The term processed foods refers to those foods that have been modified from their natural state through various methods, including refining, adding preservatives, or combining different ingredients. While processing can improve food safety, preservation for transport and shelf life and convenience, this alteration comes at a cost. The end result is ultra-processed foods that are void of important nutrients, such as fiber, vitamins, and minerals. Even fast foods, which are designed to be quickly prepared and served, are generally just high in calories, unhealthy fats, sodium, and sugar.

These ultra-processed foods are now so frequently consumed that they lead to insulin resistance, weight gain, and obesity as stored fat. This is all linked to an increased risk of type 2 diabetes, high blood pressure, heart disease, and a host of other conditions, including certain cancers.[47] Additionally, the lack of fiber in these foods can contribute to digestive problems, such as constipation, and increase the risk of colorectal cancer.

Consequences of Ultra-Processed Foods

The University of São Paulo in Brazil did a study and found that about 57,000 people died early because they ate too much ultra-processed food.[48] This made up 10.5% of all the early deaths for adults aged 30 to 69. Ultra-processed foods are between 13% to 21% of what Brazilians eat. But in America, they make up about 57% of what people eat every day, which means that more people in America might be dying because of these foods.[49] If Brazilians ate 10% to 50% less ultra-processed foods, 5,900 to 29,300 people could be saved from dying every year. And if adults ate less than 23% of ultra-processed foods every day, about 20,000 people could be saved from dying early each year.[50]

Researchers from Imperial College London's School of Public Health also found that ultra-processed foods are linked to a higher risk of developing cancer.[51] This means that if people eat more of these foods, they might get cancer more often, especially ovarian and brain cancers. Men who eat the most ultra-processed foods have a 29% higher risk of getting colorectal cancer compared to men who eat the least. These findings are so concerning that one of the researchers is calling for warning labels to be put on the packaging of these foods so people can make better choices.

Major Food Companies Best Interests

Major food corporations, such as Nestle, Pillsbury, Kraft, McDonald's, and numerous others, employ highly paid food scientists as some of their most valuable staff members. These intelligent professionals concentrate primarily on developing flavors, taste bud appeal, and other characteristics that entice consumers to consume more and more of their products. These processed food companies dedicate substantial financial resources and marketing efforts to a single objective - creating foods that stimulate a never-ending desire for more of their food.

An example of this phenomenon is wheat, which has been a nutritious staple in human diets for thousands of years. However, in the late 1800s, technological advancements enabled a more efficient grain grinding process, leading to the production of refined flour, commonly known as white flour.[52] This process stripped away the most nutrient-rich and fiber-dense parts of the grain, resulting in a less nutritious final product that is rapidly digested, causing blood sugar spikes and swift insulin responses.

Frequent consumption of foods made with refined flour can contribute to insulin resistance and a host of health issues, such as elevated blood glucose and cholesterol levels, digestive problems, and inflammation.[53] This entire situation is contributing to a health crisis. The consumption of these ultra-processed goods contributes to insulin resistance and a host of health issues, such as elevated blood glucose and cholesterol levels, digestive problems, and inflammation. As a result, prediabetes now impacts over one-third of the population, with over 84% of them being unaware of their condition.[54] Regrettably, almost half of those with prediabetes will eventually develop type 2 diabetes.[55] Although individuals need to take responsibility for their eating habits, resisting foods that are meticulously engineered to appeal to our every preference, including convenience, proves to be a challenging task.

While completely avoiding processed foods altogether may be unrealistic in today's world, we can mitigate their adverse effects by enjoying them in moderation and incorporating the many other lifestyle considerations found throughout this book. For example, fiber helps slow down the breakdown of refined grains and the absorption of glucose, ultimately supporting healthy blood sugar regulation, as well as physical exercise and other lifestyle factors.

Misleading Food Labels and Claims

Food manufacturers often use misleading language and even make false health claims on labels. This marketing tactic serves not only to sell more products but also makes it difficult for consumers to consciously select healthy options, putting them in a position of carefully examining the ingredients list. One key tip when it comes to food labels is to disregard almost all claims on the front of the packaging. Research has shown that health claims on front labels can cause consumers to perceive products as healthier, which only serves to influence their choices.[56]

Health claims on packaged food are intended to attract attention and convince you that the product is healthy.[57] While many genuinely healthy foods are organic, whole grain, or natural, the presence of such claims on a label doesn't guarantee a product's healthiness.[58]

Here are some common claims and their meanings you may find helpful:

- Light: Light products have reduced calories or fat due to processing or dilution. Check for added ingredients, like sugar, to compensate for the reduction.

- Multigrain: This simply means a product contains more

than one type of grain, which may be refined unless labeled as whole grain.

* Natural: This claim only signifies that the manufacturer used a natural source, such as apples or rice, at some stage in the process.

* Organic: This label doesn't necessarily indicate a healthy product; for instance, organic sugar is still sugar.

* No added sugar: Products can be naturally high in sugar, and unhealthy sugar substitutes might be used in place of added sugar.

* Low-calorie: These products must have one-third fewer calories than the brand's original product, but calorie counts can vary between brands.

* Low-fat: Often, fat reduction results in added sugar, so read the ingredients list carefully.

* Low-carb: Processed low-carb foods may still be unhealthy, just like processed low-fat foods.

* Made with whole grains: The product may contain minimal whole grains; check the ingredients list for whole grains within the first three ingredients.

* Fortified or enriched: Nutrients have been added to the product, but that doesn't necessarily make it healthy.

* Gluten-free: The product doesn't contain wheat, spelt, rye, or barley but can still be highly processed and full of unhealthy fats and sugar.

* Fruit-flavored: The product may not contain actual fruit,

only chemicals designed to mimic fruit flavors.

- Zero trans fat: This means less than 0.5 grams of trans fat per serving. However, if serving sizes are misleadingly small, the product could still contain trans fat.

Reading Nutrition Labels for Smart Food Choices

On the back of the packaging is where we find a detailed listing of ingredients in order of quantity, with the first ingredient often being the most abundant in the product. A helpful guideline to use is to look at the first three ingredients, as they comprise the majority of the product ingredients.

It is important to understand and use nutrition labels to our advantage in making smart food choices. Nutrition labels indicate the calories and nutrients present in a standard amount of the product, usually a suggested single serving. However, these serving sizes can be much smaller than what we typically consume in one sitting, leading to confusion about the actual contents of the product.

To begin, it is best to narrow your focus, it is helpful to pay attention to serving size, sodium, and carbohydrates (specifically fiber and sugar), and gradually expand the information you look at such as the fat (trans fats) and protein.

Those who follow a keto or low carb diet, or who have diabetes, often count the amount of carbs in their diet. In many cases, calculating net carbs is a better formula to follow and to understand the total carbs in the food. Start by looking at the total carbs on the nutrition label. Then look at the total sugars, which is often sugar that is included as part of the food or added. Then look at the amount of fiber. To calculate net carbs take the carbs and the fiber. Keeping in mind that for every 4g of net carbs in the food, from a glucose impact standpoint, it is like eating 1 teaspoon of sugar. Increasing the intake of dietary fiber and decreasing the intake of total net carbs and added sugar is always beneficial.

Nutrition Facts Valeur nutritive Per 1 cup (250 mL) / par 1 tasse (250 mL)	
Amount / Teneur	% Daily Value / % valeur quotidienne
Calories / Calories 80	
Fat / Lipides 0 g	0 %
Saturated / saturés 0 g + Trans / trans 0 g	0 %
Cholesterol / Cholestérol 0 mg	
Sodium / Sodium 115 mg	5 %
Carbohydrate / Glucides 12 g	4 %
Fibre / Fibres 0 g	0 %
Sugars / Sucres 11 g	
Protein / Protéines 9 g	
Vitamin A / Vitamine A	15 %
Vitamin C / Vitamine C	0 %
Calcium / Calcium	30 %
Iron / Fer	0 %
Vitamin D / Vitamine D	45 %

When you read and understand nutrition labels, you'll know more about which "other ingredients" are added for the food's taste, texture, appearance, and shelf life. These may include sodium, sweeteners, preservatives, trans fats, as well as refined sugars and grains.

By learning about serving sizes, calories, fats, sodium, carbohydrates, protein, and other important ingredients on the label, we can be empowered to make better dietary decisions. Scientific research shows that paying attention to nutrition labels can result in a higher intake of fiber, calcium, and vitamin C, and a lower intake of calories and carbohydrates.[59]

Although it may seem confusing at first, practicing reading nutrition labels can make it easier over time, enabling you to make the most of every bite. Remember, nutrition labels are a valuable tool for reaching long-term goals and maintaining a healthy lifestyle.

Choosing Whole, Healthy Foods

When it comes to food, unfortunately as a society we value convenience and speed over nutrition and long term health. But the negative effects of these decisions compounded over time are clear, as we can see in the growing number of chronic health issues.

The answer is to focus more on eating whole, healthy foods that are lower on the glycemic index. This means choosing fresh fruits and vegetables, lean proteins, and whole grains instead of processed and fast foods. Generally, avoiding fast foods that are highly processed and those made in factories that come in boxes, bags, and barcodes will always serve you best.

A good first step is to read food labels carefully and know what we're eating. Choose whole foods that aren't heavily processed and avoid those high in sugar, salt, and unhealthy fats, which can make a significant difference in our health. A second step is to increase dietary fiber through food intake and incorporate the *fiber matrix drink* that can be found at beyondfeelgreatbook.com.

It's essential to pay attention to our food choices and put more effort into choosing whole, healthy foods over processed and fast foods. By making this change, as well as adding more fiber with meals, we can improve our health and avoid many problems linked to the modern food world.

$\underline{ella}$

Insulin Resistance: The Impact on Health

Now that we have covered the glucose-insulin cycle, as well as the impact of the food we eat and the modern food environment we live in, in this chapter, we will take a deeper look into insulin resistance and why it is so important to understand.

Insulin is a hormone produced by the pancreas that helps regulate glucose, or blood sugar levels. Glucose is an important source of energy for our bodies, fueling our cells and supporting bodily functions. The food we eat is broken down into proteins, fats, and carbohydrates, which are then used in metabolism or cell replacement. The amount of fuel our bodies need varies, but our blood sugar levels must remain stable. Insulin plays a crucial role in this process by signaling the body's cells to absorb glucose from the bloodstream and use it for energy or storage.

Ideally, glucose is carried in the bloodstream to individual cells, where insulin signals the cells to absorb the glucose and use it for energy or storage. However, when there is too much glucose in the body, cells can become desensitized to insulin, which can lead to insulin resistance. In response, the body may continue to release more insulin, seeking to lower the blood sugar levels.

Insulin resistance occurs when cells of the body no longer respond to insulin in the same way they used to.[60] This can happen in fat and muscle cells, as well as in other cells throughout the body that have insulin receptors. Insulin receptors are found in cells such as nerves, blood cells, bones, and others. Each of these cells has different responses to insulin, but the common theme is that insulin is telling the cells to grow.

Insulin resistance affects all cells and can lead to the development of numerous conditions associated with diabetes, such as neuropathy. It's important to note, however, that these conditions aren't solely caused by glucose levels. Rather, they can begin to manifest even before glucose levels change, because insulin plays a key role in driving these health issues.[61]

Insulin resistance occurs when cells in the muscles, body fat, and liver no longer respond to insulin's signal to absorb glucose from the bloodstream and use it for energy or storage. Glucose, also known as blood sugar, is one of the body's primary sources of fuel.

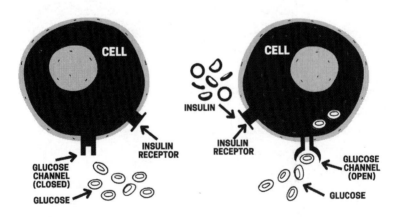

While genetics, aging, and ethnicity play roles in developing insulin sensitivity, the driving forces behind insulin resistance include dietary lifestyle resulting in excess body weight, too much belly fat, a lack of exercise, smoking, and even lack of adequate sleep plays a role.

As insulin resistance develops, your body fights back by producing more insulin. Over months and years, the beta cells in your pancreas that are working so hard to make insulin get worn out and can no longer keep pace with the demand for more and more insulin. Then, after years of this, insulin resistance silently begins and blood sugar continues to rise, and many develop prediabetes and then type 2 diabetes. Some may also develop non-alcoholic fatty liver disease, a growing problem associated with insulin resistance that increases the risk for liver damage and heart disease.[62]

Insulin resistance can also lead to high levels of triglycerides and LDL (bad) cholesterol in the blood, as well as high blood pressure, increasing the risk of heart disease.

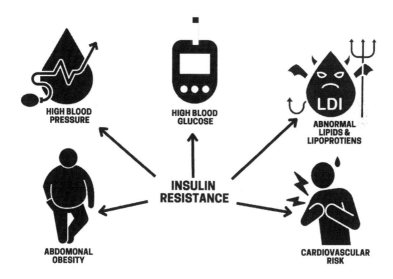

Dr. Ben Bikman, in his book, *Insulin Resistance*, stated that almost every chronic disease, to some degree, is going to be either caused by, or made worse by, insulin resistance.[63]

Dr. Bikman has also claimed that Alzheimer's disease, migraines, fatty liver disease, hypertension, osteoarthritis, and many other conditions are linked to insulin resistance. In women, conditions such as polycystic ovarian syndrome (PCOS) can also be associated with insulin resistance. Despite the apparent lack of connection between these conditions, insulin resistance is often the underlying cause.[64]

Reversing insulin resistance requires making changes to your diet and lifestyle. Fiber becomes a crucial nutrient that plays a significant role in managing insulin resistance. Soluble fiber forms a gel-like substance in the digestive system, slowing down glucose absorption into the bloodstream. This helps prevent blood sugar spikes and crashes, which can contribute to insulin resistance over time. That's where the *fiber matrix drink* comes in - as its a science-based, fiber-rich supplement that can be an effective strategy for managing insulin resistance and promoting overall health.

Fiber may also positively affect the gut microbiome, influencing insulin sensitivity. Research shows that individuals with insulin resistance tend to have less diverse gut microbiomes, and increasing fiber intake may promote a healthier, more diverse microbiome.[65]

This book provides you with essential principles to overcome and reduce insulin resistance. By applying these principles, such as incorporating the *fiber matrix drink* into your routine and following the Glycemic Index as outlined in the *Food Guide*, you can take control of your health and experience lasting improvements. For more information and to access these resources, please visit beyondfeelgreatbook.com.

Chapter 6

Leptin & Ghrelin Resistance: The Disconnect

Leptin was first discovered in 1994. It's a hormone produced by fat cells that regulates appetite and metabolism, signaling the brain when the body has enough nourishment, prompting it to stop eating, and helping to maintain a healthy body weight. Leptin also supports efficient metabolism.

Leptin travels through your blood, via your circulatory system, to the appetite center of your brain. There, it binds to receptors that are responsible for making you feel hungry. Leptin also travels through the nervous system, stimulating fatty tissue to burn off fat and calories.

When too much leptin builds up in the blood, we can develop leptin resistance. In cases of leptin resistance, the brain does not respond to leptin as it typically should. As a result, nothing prevents us from experiencing the sensation of fullness or satiety, leading us to eat more food even though our body already has sufficient fat stores.[66]

As a result, your body thinks it's starving and slows down your metabolism (how fast you burn calories) to conserve energy. This makes it easier to gain weight and harder to lose it. Your body also tends to store more fat instead of burning it for energy, which can make you gain even more weight over time.

So, in short, leptin resistance can make you feel hungry all the time, slow down your metabolism, and promote weight gain. Over time, the brain may become desensitized to leptin, leading to overeating, weight gain, and an increased risk of chronic diseases such as type 2 diabetes, heart disease, and certain cancers.[67]

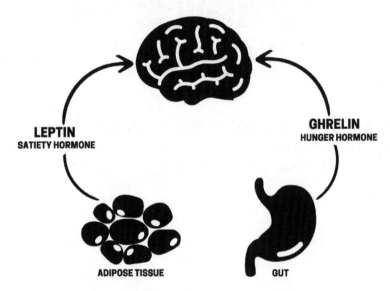

Ghrelin, on the other side, is a hormone responsible for boosting appetite. It is secreted by the stomach when it is empty, signaling the brain that it's time for a meal.[68] Ghrelin acts quickly and should decrease substantially once you're full. Its levels reach their peak just before eating and drop to their lowest point about an hour after consumption, remaining low for approximately three hours.

Research suggests that ghrelin levels in individuals with obesity decline only marginally after eating. This can cause the brain to assume that additional food is necessary, potentially resulting in overeating.[69]

The understanding of the underlying causes of leptin and ghrelin resistance is crucial for effectively addressing these issues. One primary cause of leptin resistance is chronic inflammation. Inflammatory signals in the hypothalamus, the brain region responsible for regulating appetite and energy balance, can impair the brain's ability to detect and respond to leptin. This inflammation can arise from various sources, including poor diet, lack of physical activity, and obesity itself. High levels of circulating leptin due to excessive fat stores can also contribute to resistance, as the brain becomes desensitized to the hormone's signaling.

Another factor contributing to leptin resistance is the disruption of the blood-brain barrier. This barrier is responsible for regulating the passage of molecules, including hormones, between the bloodstream and the brain. In some cases, obesity can compromise the blood-brain barrier's integrity, hindering leptin from reaching the hypothalamus and thereby reducing its effectiveness in signaling satiety.

Ghrelin resistance is less well understood, but is believed to be influenced by similar factors. Chronic inflammation, poor diet, and obesity can contribute to alterations in ghrelin signaling.[70] In individuals with obesity, ghrelin levels may not decrease effectively after eating, leading to persistent hunger and overeating. Inadequate sleep can increase ghrelin levels, promoting hunger and overeating, while also reducing leptin levels, further disrupting the balance between hunger and satiety signals.

Addressing the underlying causes of leptin and ghrelin resistance requires making changes to your diet and lifestyle including increasing physical activity, reducing inflammation, managing stress levels, and ensuring adequate sleep.

By adopting these healthier lifestyle habits and addressing these root causes, we can restore the natural balance of these essential

hormones and work towards achieving and maintaining our
health as it was intended.[71]

Addressing leptin resistance requires making changes to your diet
and lifestyle. Fiber, from foods as well as the *fiber matrix drink*,
plays a significant role in managing leptin resistance. By promoting
satiety, supporting gut health, and regulating blood sugar levels,
fiber can have a positive impact on leptin and ghrelin resistance.[72]

Fiber plays a vital role in supporting healthy digestion and overall
well-being and can help manage leptin and ghrelin resistance. The
relationship between fiber and these appetite-regulating hormones
is primarily due to the effects of fiber on satiety, gut health, and
blood sugar regulation.

Fiber, particularly soluble fiber, can slow down the absorption
of glucose into the bloodstream, preventing rapid fluctuations
in blood sugar levels. Stable blood sugar levels help maintain
consistent energy levels and prevent insulin resistance, which is
often associated with leptin resistance .[73]

By applying these principles, such as using the *fiber matrix drink*,
incorporating high-fiber foods, and focusing on low glycemic
foods as listed in the *Food Guide*, you'll be able to take control of
your health and achieve lasting improvements in your well-being.
To download the *Food Guide* and learn more about the *fiber
matrix drink*, visit beyondfeelgreatbook.com.

Chapter 7

Blood Pressure and Insulin: The Connection

Hypertension is a major health concern with sometimes devastating consequences. High blood pressure and insulin resistance are interconnected health conditions that can lead to serious health problems, such as heart disease, stroke, and kidney disease.[74]

As discussed in previous chapters, insulin resistance occurs when cells become less responsive to insulin, resulting in elevated insulin and glucose levels in the blood. Over time, this can damage blood vessels and increase the risk of high blood pressure. High blood pressure, in contrast, arises when the force of blood against arterial walls is consistently too high, causing harm to blood vessels and organs.

High blood pressure, also known as hypertension, is often referred to as a "silent killer" because it typically presents no noticeable symptoms in its early stages. As a result, many people are unaware they have the condition until complications arise. However, in some cases, symptoms may manifest, including severe headaches, dizziness, shortness of breath, blurred vision, chest pain, or nosebleeds.

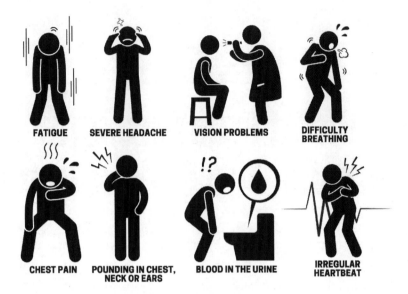

FATIGUE   SEVERE HEADACHE   VISION PROBLEMS   DIFFICULTY BREATHING

CHEST PAIN   POUNDING IN CHEST, NECK OR EARS   BLOOD IN THE URINE   IRREGULAR HEARTBEAT

The connection between insulin resistance and high blood pressure is complex, but several mechanisms can help explain the connection.

One critical factor is insulin's role in regulating sodium reabsorption in the kidneys. When cells become resistant to insulin, the kidneys may reabsorb excessive sodium, increasing blood volume and leading to higher blood pressure. Insulin resistance can also result in the production of reactive oxygen species, causing inflammation and damage to blood vessels and contributing to the development of atherosclerosis.[75]

Other factors linking insulin resistance and high blood pressure include obesity, physical inactivity, and a diet high in processed foods and sugar. These factors increase the risk of both conditions and contribute to metabolic syndrome development, characterized by a cluster of health issues, including high blood pressure, high blood sugar levels, and excess body fat around the waist.

Recognizing this connection between insulin resistance and high blood pressure is vital for devising effective prevention and management strategies. By reducing the risk of both conditions, individuals can improve their overall health and decrease the likelihood of long-term complications, including heart disease, stroke, and kidney disease. Prioritizing healthy lifestyle habits and collaborating with healthcare providers to manage these conditions is essential for promoting long-term health.

Insulin resistance is a health condition that arises when the body's cells do not respond effectively to insulin, a hormone that regulates blood sugar levels. Consequently, the body produces more insulin to lower blood sugar levels, leading to higher than normal insulin levels in the bloodstream. Elevated insulin levels can contribute to high blood pressure development, as extra insulin can constrict blood vessels and increase their resistance to blood flow. Additionally, high blood sugar levels can damage blood vessels, increasing the risk of hypertension by causing the vessels to become stiff and narrow.

Lowering Blood Pressure Naturally

Managing blood pressure and insulin resistance requires a comprehensive approach involving lifestyle changes and, if necessary, medication. Although medications are often prescribed as the first line of treatment for lowering blood pressure, there is not enough emphasis on addressing insulin resistance. It is crucial to understand that insulin resistance and cardiovascular disorders are closely linked.

Maintaining a healthy weight, engaging in regular physical activity, and following a healthy diet are all crucial strategies for reducing the risk of these conditions. Additionally, reducing sodium intake, avoiding processed foods and added sugars, and consuming a fiber-rich diet can help lower blood pressure and improve insulin sensitivity.

A fiber-rich diet has numerous health benefits, including lowering high blood pressure. Soluble fiber, found in foods such as oats, barley, beans, and certain fruits and vegetables, can reduce blood pressure by binding to cholesterol in the digestive system and facilitating its removal from the body. This process reduces low-density lipoprotein (LDL) cholesterol, which contributes to atherosclerosis – a condition characterized by plaque accumulation in the arteries that causes them to narrow and raises blood pressure.

Fiber also helps maintain a healthy body weight by promoting satiety, reducing overall caloric intake, and supporting a healthy gut microbiome. Since obesity is a major risk factor for hypertension, a fiber-rich diet can help prevent and manage high blood pressure. Incorporating a variety of fiber-rich foods, such as whole grains, fruits, vegetables, legumes, and nuts, into your daily diet can improve cardiovascular health and reduce the risk of hypertension.

In conclusion, insulin resistance and high blood sugar levels can contribute to hypertension by damaging blood vessels and increasing insulin production in the body. By maintaining healthy blood sugar levels and managing insulin resistance through dietary and lifestyle changes, individuals can reduce the risk of developing hypertension.[76]

A key challenge is consuming enough dietary fiber through food intake while maintaining a healthy routine and overcoming unhealthy habits and cravings. This is where the *fiber matrix drink* can be invaluable in reducing insulin resistance and lowering blood pressure. To learn more visit beyondfeelgreatbook.com.

Chapter 8

Metabolic Flexibility: The Energy Switch

The human body is a remarkable system that requires energy to function, and the food we eat provides that energy. Our food is composed of three primary macronutrients: protein, carbohydrate, and fat. Our bodies are designed to use both carbohydrates and fats for energy, and we call this ability to switch between these macronutrients—metabolic flexibility.

This ability has magnificently served us throughout history in times of surplus when food was plentiful, and in times of famine when food was scarce. However, due to the way we eat today, most of us find ourselves perpetually in a surplus state of having carbohydrate glucose energy. As a result, we have become better at storing energy than using it, leading to a dramatic increase in poor metabolic health worldwide.

The term "metabolic health" has been gaining popularity, but its meaning and significance may not be clear to everyone. This chapter aims to explore the concept of metabolic health to give a better connection to our overall health and well-being.

Metabolic health can be viewed as an umbrella term, when using the term 'metabolic syndrome' it is often used to identify a range of conditions such as obesity, type 2 diabetes and heart disease, and when using the term metabolic health it can also define a life without these conditions. Achieving optimal metabolic health is often referred to as being in a state where we can maintain a healthy waist circumference, blood sugars, blood pressure, cholesterol, and triglycerides—this leads to having abundant energy and focus, and living a healthy fulfilling life without chronic disease. According to a 2019 study in the journal Metabolic Health and Related Disorders, only 12 percent of American adults are considered metabolically healthy.[77]

To attain optimal metabolic health, it is crucial to focus on metabolic flexibility. Our bodies require energy to function, and this energy is derived from both carbohydrates and fats. Metabolic flexibility refers to the body's ability to efficiently switch between utilizing both carbohydrates and fats as energy sources, allowing us to have adequate energy to power our bodily functions and burn the fuel it prefers, whether we're lounging on the couch or exercising at the gym.

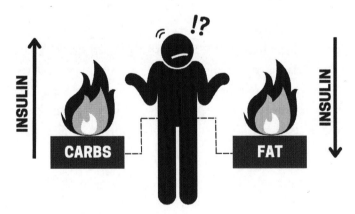

Metabolic efficiency is another critical aspect of metabolic health. An efficient metabolism burns the calories consumed, reducing the need to store excess calories. This is vital because an inefficient metabolism can lead to the accumulation of extra calories, which can contribute to weight gain and other chronic health issues.

Metabolic inflexibility can be caused by several factors, including a diet high in processed foods and sugar, a sedentary lifestyle, chronic stress, and poor sleep habits. Consuming a diet that is high in processed foods and sugar can lead to insulin resistance, which reduces the body's ability to utilize carbohydrates as energy. This can result in the body relying more on carbs as a fuel source, which leads to metabolic inflexibility.

Metabolic flexibility is a vital aspect of our overall health and well-being that can be improved by implementing various lifestyle changes. Time-restricted eating and intermittent fasting are effective methods for enhancing metabolic flexibility. During intermittent fasting, the body uses carbohydrates before switching to fat stores, which can help train metabolic flexibility. Low to moderate-intensity exercise while in a fasted state, can also help improve metabolic flexibility and enhance overall metabolism.

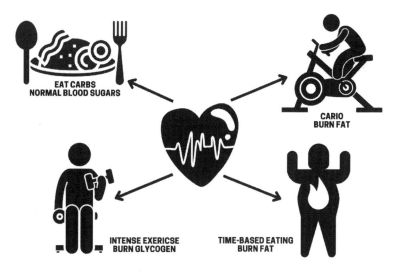

Engaging in regular physical activity is another important factor in controlling insulin levels and promoting metabolic flexibility. Exercise stimulates glucose uptake into our muscles, reducing the amount of glucose in the bloodstream and lowering insulin levels.

This will help the body improve insulin sensitivity and help the body to use stored fat for energy.

Reducing chronic inflammation is also crucial for optimizing metabolic health. Poor diet, stress, lack of sleep, and environmental toxins can cause chronic inflammation, impairing insulin sensitivity, leading to metabolic dysfunction. Consuming low glycemic anti-inflammatory foods, such as leafy greens, fatty fish, nuts, seeds, and olive oil, can help reduce inflammation and improve metabolic flexibility. Stress reduction techniques like meditation, yoga, and deep breathing can also help reduce inflammation and improve overall metabolic function.

Understanding and implementing metabolic flexibility can greatly improve one's overall health and well-being. By taking small steps towards optimizing our metabolism, we can reap the numerous benefits that come with it. If you want to learn more about metabolic flexibility and other strategies for achieving optimal health, visit beyondfeelgreatbook.com for further resources and information.

Chapter 9

Intermittent Fasting: Basics & Benefits

Intermittent fasting, or time-restricted eating, is a dietary approach that has been gaining popularity in recent years due to its potential health benefits. By restricting calorie intake for a certain period of time, this method allows the body to enter a fasted state, which has been associated with a number of positive health benefits.

Intermittent fasting has become popular dietary approach. Because of its many health benefits. This eating pattern involves switching between periods of eating and not eating, which can last a few hours or in some cases a whole day. Intermittent fasting can help with weight loss by cutting down the total amount of food you eat and increasing how fast your body burns calories. This makes it helpful for people who want to reach or maintain a healthy weight.

The Health Benefits

Intermittent fasting can also help the body control blood sugars and use insulin better, which improves insulin sensitivity, and reduces the risk of type 2 diabetes.[78] It's good for your heart too, as it can lower blood pressure, cholesterol levels, and inflammation. Another benefit is that intermittent fasting helps your body repair and remove damaged cells, promoting overall health and a longer life. By adding intermittent fasting to a well-balanced lifestyle, people can enjoy a variety of health benefits and lower the risk of different long-term health concerns.[79]

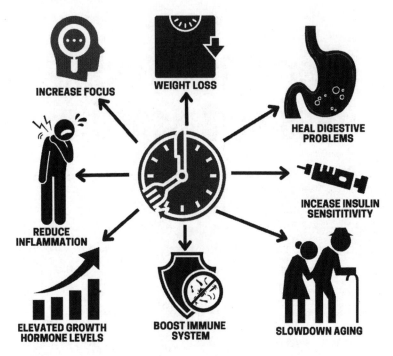

Intermittent fasting is a simple eating pattern where you switch between a time-based routine of eating and not eating. Generally, intermittent fasting itself is not about what foods you eat, but when you eat them. With intermittent fasting, you might skip breakfast, eat only during certain hours of the day, or avoid food for a whole day once or twice a week. By doing this, you naturally eat less, give your body a break from digesting food, and allow it to focus on other important functions, like repairing cells and using stored energy. Many people find intermittent fasting easier to follow than restrictive diets, and it can lead to various health benefits like better weight management, improved blood sugar control, and a healthier heart.

A Natural Addition: Yerba Mate

In recent years people are discovering that incorporating yerba mate into a morning fasting period offers many benefits.[80] Yerba mate is a plant native to South America, traditionally consumed as a tea, and is known for its natural energy-boosting and antioxidant properties. By integrating this drink into their fasting routine, it's proven that you will experience increased energy levels, heightened mental clarity, and improved focus without the need for calorie-dense breakfasts or high-sugar beverages. Additionally, the antioxidants in yerba mate can help combat free radicals, reducing inflammation and supporting overall health.

Most importantly for intermittent fasting, yerba mate has been shown to possess appetite-suppressing qualities so it doesn't feel like fasting is starving yourself. A study published in the Journal Nutrients in 2015 found that yerba mate consumption can increase GLP-1 levels, which can help improve insulin sensitivity and reduce appetite.[81]

GLP-1 is a hormone that our body makes in the gut when we eat. It helps control our blood sugar levels by telling our pancreas to release insulin, which lowers the amount of sugar in our blood. GLP-1 also slows down how quickly food is absorbed into our body, which further helps control blood sugar levels.

Apart from controlling blood sugar, GLP-1 also helps us lose weight, reduce inflammation, and improve our heart health. Doctors sometimes use GLP-1 drugs to treat people with type 2 diabetes or obesity because of these benefits.

Semaglutide is a type 2 diabetes drug sold under the brand names Ozempic and Wegovy. It is also used as a weight loss treatment and has become popular among celebrities because it works similarly to GLP-1, another hormone that helps control blood sugar levels and promotes weight loss. Yerba mate has been clinically proven to be a natural alternative to semaglutide.

A study published in the journal Nutrients in 2017 found that the combination of yerba mate consumption and exercise enhances mood states and improves control over satiety and appetite - key elements for a lifestyle optimized for metabolic health and fat loss.[82] This is just one of many studies indicating that yerba mate may increase the body's production of GLP-1. Researchers are actively investigating the mechanisms underlying this unique effect of yerba mate.

There is a wide array of yerba mate brands available in the market, each varying in quality and price point. My go-to choice is an ultra-concentrated, on-the-go *yerba mate drink* conveniently packaged in single-serving packets. Backed by science, this drink provides a natural kickstart to the day and aids in weight control by curbing the urge to snack between meals. It serves as an excellent tool for enhancing the overall experience of intermittent fasting.

If you want to learn more about the benefits and science behind yerba mate, check out the resource page for this book beyondfeelgreatbook.com for more information. You'll discover that yerba mate is an excellent source of naturally occurring caffeine and other health-promoting compounds, making it a convenient and effective way to boost energy levels and improve mental clarity throughout the day.

It's important to underscore that intermittent fasting is not about starving oneself, demonizing food, or using the practice as an excuse to binge eat during meal times. Rather, intermittent fasting is a method that provides your body with a break from digestion, allowing it to focus on other essential bodily processes.

Breaking a Fast: The debate and the nuances

One of the most confusing aspects of intermittent fasting is what actually 'breaks a fast'. In general, any calorie intake is considered breaking a fast, but opinions vary among nutritional experts on the number of calories needed for a fast to be broken.[83] Some experts recommend sticking to a zero-calorie and carbohydrate rule during the fasting period to ensure that the fast is not broken. This means avoiding all forms of food, drinks, or supplements that contain calories or carbohydrates.

However, the body's physiological processes during fasting are not a simple on/off switch. There are degrees of fasting, and the impact of a small number of calories on a fast may vary depending on the individual, the length of the fast and the overall health goals.[84]

Coffee While Fasting

The question of whether or not it is okay to have coffee during a fasting period is a common one. In general, drinking black coffee is fine and has several potential health benefits. Caffeine, a natural stimulant found in coffee, can increase energy levels and improve physical and cognitive performance. Additionally, coffee consumption has been linked to a reduced risk of developing certain diseases such as type 2 diabetes, liver disease, and Parkinson's disease.

When it comes to fasting, drinking black coffee is generally considered safe because it contains very few calories, usually less than 5 calories per 8-ounce serving. This low-calorie content makes black coffee a good choice for those who want to enjoy a cup of coffee during their fasting period without breaking their fast. However, it is important to keep in mind that the calorie (carb) content of coffee can quickly increase if you add sugar, milk, cream, or other sweeteners to your coffee. So, if you are trying not to break your fasting period, it is important to be mindful of your coffee choices.

One reason that black coffee is often considered safe during fasting is that caffeine can increase the production of a chemical called cAMP. This chemical activates a protein called AMPK, which helps the body break down stored glycogen and fats for energy. AMPK is an important enzyme that helps regulate energy use in the body, and it is activated during fasting to help increase energy production and decrease energy consumption.[85]

It's worth noting that if you are drinking coffee and not seeing the results you want from your intermittent fasting routine, it may be worth considering reducing or eliminating your coffee intake to see if that helps. In some cases, caffeine intake may negatively impact fasting benefits, so it is important to pay attention to your body's response.

Guidelines for Breaking a Fast

When breaking a fast, it is important to choose foods that are low on the glycemic index, high in fiber and protein, and rich in healthy fats. Avoiding foods with added sugars and saturated fats and staying away from processed foods is also beneficial. It is important to break your fast with a nutrient-dense meal that will help replenish your body with essential nutrients and provide sustained energy for the rest of the day.

Here are some guidelines for choosing the best foods to eat when breaking a fast:

- Focus on Protein: Eating protein-rich foods can help you feel fuller and more satisfied, which can help you avoid overeating. Good sources of protein include eggs, lean meats, poultry, fish, beans, and lentils.

- Choose Low GI Foods: When breaking a fast, it is

important to focus on low glycemic, unprocessed foods. This means choosing fresh fruits and vegetables, whole grains, and nuts and seeds. Avoid packaged and processed foods, which can be high in added sugars, salt, and unhealthy fats.

• Incorporate Healthy Fats: Including healthy fats in your meals can help you feel fuller and more satisfied, while also providing important nutrients for your body. Good sources of healthy fats include avocados, nuts and seeds, olive oil, and fatty fish like salmon.

• Avoid Sugary Foods: Consuming sugary foods can cause a spike in your blood sugar levels, which can lead to a crash and leave you feeling sluggish. Instead, choose natural sweeteners like honey, maple syrup, or dates in moderation.

• Stay Hydrated: When breaking a fast, it is important to drink plenty of water to help flush toxins from your body and keep you hydrated. You can also drink herbal tea, coconut water, or bone broth to replenish electrolytes and other nutrients.

Overall, it is important to be mindful of your food choices when breaking a fast to maximize the benefits of your fast and maintain a healthy and balanced diet.

Intermittent Fasting and COVID-19: A Possible Connection

Although the reason for the link between intermittent fasting and better COVID-19 outcomes is not yet fully understood, research has shown that fasting helps reduce inflammation by lowering the number of pro-inflammatory cells in the blood and can trigger autophagy, which is the process by which the body breaks down old and damaged cells.[86]

An interesting study showed that those who regularly practiced intermittent fasting as a lifestyle routine prior to the pandemic, had a lower risk of hospitalization and mortality from COVID-19, and could prevent infection.[87]

Other studies have shown that severe COVID-19 cases are typically associated with cardiometabolic health issues, such as type 2 diabetes, insulin resistance, and cardiovascular disease.[88] While fasting is not a cure-all, the study's authors believe that it may improve cardiometabolic health and may limit COVID-19 severity. In another study, it was found that those who practiced regular intermittent fasting were less likely to be hospitalized or die from COVID-19 than those who did not follow the eating plan.[89]

Enhancing the Fasting Experience

Intermittent fasting offers a powerful dietary approach with numerous health benefits, including enhanced insulin sensitivity, fat burning, and reduced risk of chronic diseases.

Incorporating the *yerba mate drink* during fasting can make the experience more comfortable by providing natural energy, mental clarity, and appetite suppression without disrupting the fasting state. It is worth noting that the effect of a minimal number of calories on fasting may vary from person to person.

Understanding the fundamentals of intermittent fasting and the benefits of yerba mate can help you make well-informed choices about its suitability for you and implement it safely and effectively for optimal results.

Chapter 10

Macro & Micro Nutrients: The Keys

It's not just what you eat; it's also what you're not eating in your foods. In the previous chapters, we covered ultra-processed foods. There are four macronutrients; 16 vitamins; 60 minerals; and three oils. In this chapter, we will go through each of these categories and explain them in more detail as we need these for optimum health.

Proper nutrition is essential for good health, and the nutrients we consume play a critical role in maintaining our overall well-being. Among the many nutrients our bodies require, macro and micro nutrients are particularly important. Macro nutrients, such as carbohydrates, proteins, and fats, provide us with the energy we need to carry out our daily activities; while micro nutrients, such as vitamins and minerals, play a key role in supporting our immune system, regulating our metabolism, and ensuring healthy growth and development.

Macronutrients are the essential nutrients required by the body in larger quantities to support various bodily functions such as growth, repair, and energy production. It is important to consume a balanced diet that includes all three macronutrients in appropriate proportions to ensure the body has the necessary nutrients to function optimally. There are three primary macronutrients:

Carbohydrates: Finding the Right Balance

Carbohydrates have become the body's primary source of energy as a result of today's modern food environment. Foods supply carbohydrates in three forms: starch, sugar, and cellulose (fiber). Today, most people consume around half of their diet as carbohydrates. This often comes from rice, wheat, bread, potatoes, pasta, and other carbs.

When it comes to improving health, finding the right amount and type of carbohydrates is essential. While carbohydrates are not an 'essential nutrient', they are still found in healthy foods that provide tremendous value to our metabolic health. In the past, carbohydrates were often viewed negatively, as well; dietary fat was considered a macronutrient to severely limit or avoid because it could make you fat. However, with expanding research into how food affects the human body, we now know that dietary fat is beneficial in a variety of cases. Similarly, carbohydrates serve an important role in normal human functioning, and no one macronutrient is more important than another. We need all of them for optimum metabolic health.

Low carb diets for weight loss have become popular for their ability to shed pounds fast. One example is the Ketogenic (Keto) diet, which has been well-documented for its benefits. A traditional keto diet involves consuming about 5% carbohydrates, 20% protein, and 75% fat, while the Atkins diet, for example, focuses on eating as much fat and protein as possible while avoiding carbs. However, these diets are often adopted strictly for short-term weight loss goals, without considering other health metabolic factors.

Many people adopt the ketogenic diet for the high protein and fat intake, and the ability to lose weight quickly. However, not all protein and fats are created equal, and many people end up consuming mostly unhealthy sources, offering very little of the essential amino and fatty acids needed for good health. Eating a diet high in processed fatty foods without understanding the differences may result in a temporary 'outer appearance' of weight loss, but it can put individuals at risk of developing insulin resistance and other conditions connected to metabolic syndrome in the long term.

To improve metabolic health, it is important to focus on eliminating major sources of high glycemic foods, and to focus more on low and medium glycemic foods. For a full listing of these foods download the *Food Guide*. listing the Foods to Avoid (high GI), Foods in Moderation (medium GI), and Foods to Enjoy (low GI), at beyondfeelgreatbook.com.

Fiber: A Key for Health

Fiber is considered a macronutrient, which is a type of carbohydrate. There are two types of fiber, soluble and insoluble. Unlike other carbohydrates such as sugars and starches, fiber is not digested or absorbed in the small intestine. Instead, it passes through the digestive system relatively intact, providing various health benefits. Soluble fiber dissolves in water and can help lower cholesterol levels, while insoluble fiber does not dissolve in water and helps regulate bowel movements and promote feelings of fullness.

Fiber intake is closely tied to metabolic health. And most Americans aren't eating enough of it. According to the USDA Dietary Guidelines, dietary fiber is a dietary component of public health concern with "more than 90 percent of women and 97 percent of men do not meet recommended intakes for dietary fiber," in part because more than 85 percent of adults don't eat enough fruits, vegetables, and whole grains.[90] What's worse, their recommendations for 30 grams per day may be lower than we really need for optimal health, which is closer to 50 grams or more.

Fiber is a type of carbohydrate found in plant-based foods, such as fruits, vegetables, whole grains, and legumes. It is classified into two types: soluble and insoluble. Soluble fiber can help lower cholesterol, blood sugar, and insulin, prevent cancer, balance hormone levels, remove excess estrogen and reduce the risk of breast cancer, make vitamins and minerals, provide food for the colon cells, and more. Insoluble fiber adds bulk to the stool, promoting regular bowel movements and preventing constipation.

Fiber also helps with satiety, keeping you full after a meal because of how it slows the digestion process. Research shows that fiber can lower blood sugar as much as some diabetes medications, lower cholesterol, and promote weight loss. A 2001 study in the journal Nutrition Reviews found that people with diabetes who ate 50 grams of dietary fiber a day for six weeks had better lipid and blood glucose profiles than those who ate only 25 grams per day.[91] The American Dietetic Association has even recommended that individuals with diabetes should consume 30 to 50 grams per day to promote lower blood sugars.

Keep in mind that for some people, suddenly increasing fiber intake can cause gastrointestinal problems like indigestion, bloating, and constipation, so it is important to increase fiber intake slowly to allow the body to adjust.

Incorporating fiber-rich foods in your diet is essential for maintaining optimal health. However, it can be challenging to consume the recommended daily amount of fiber through food alone. That's where the *fiber matrix drink* comes in handy. It's an excellent way to add soluble and insoluble fiber to your daily intake while also lowering the glycemic impact of the carbohydrates in your meal. To learn more about the *fiber matrix drink* and how it can help you improve your health, visit beyondfeelgreatbook.com.

Protein: Vital for Optimal Health

Protein is essential for building and repairing tissues, as well as for various bodily functions. Proteins are the main tissue builders in the body, they are part of every cell in the body. Proteins help in cell structure, functions, hemoglobin formation to carry oxygen, manufacture enzymes to carry out vital reactions, and many other functions in the body. Proteins are necessary for nutrition because they contain amino acids. Among the amino acids, we need the eight essential amino acids from food sources, these include: lysine, tryptophan, methionine, leucine, isoleucine, phenylalanine, valine, and threonine. Foods like meat, fish, eggs, and beans are good sources of protein.

Protein is a vital macronutrient that is often overlooked, but it plays a critical role in maintaining overall health and well-being. It is a building block for the body's tissues, and it aids in the maintenance and repair of cells. While fiber often receives attention for its role in weight loss and blood sugar management, protein is equally important for these goals.

Eating enough protein is essential for staying full, reducing blood sugar spikes, burning more calories, building muscle, and recovering after exercise. On the other hand, not consuming enough protein can lead to increased hunger, consuming more calories, blood sugar highs and lows, losing more muscle mass when losing weight, and having more cravings.

Increasing protein intake is a helpful tool for making weight loss easier. Studies have shown that a higher percentage of protein in the diet is an effective way to lose weight and feel less hungry. Eating a high protein breakfast is especially helpful in promoting weight loss and preventing overeating throughout the day.

Protein can also help preserve muscle mass during weight loss, which is essential for maintaining a healthy metabolism and promoting weight loss. In addition to supporting weight loss, protein also helps regulate blood sugar levels, which is particularly important for people with type 2 diabetes.

It is recommended to consume 0.8 grams of protein per kilogram of body weight per day, although the latest research suggests a minimum of about 1.2 grams per kilogram of body weight (0.54 grams/pound) per day is best. Athletes and the elderly could benefit from consuming even more protein, at around 1.6 grams/kilogram (0.71 grams/pound) per day.[92]

There are many sources of dietary protein, including animal-based and plant-based options. Quality protein sources include lean meats, fish, poultry, eggs, beans, legumes, peas, soy, nuts, seeds, and whole grains like quinoa. It is important to choose healthy protein sources and to avoid unhealthy options, such as processed meats, fried proteins, and highly processed protein bars and shakes.

Protein shakes can be a convenient way to supplement daily protein intake and make it easier to reach protein goals, although it is important to choose high-quality protein powders that do not contain added sugars or unhealthy additives. For guidelines on choosing protein shake powders, visit beyondfeelgreatbook.com.

Protein is also helpful for those practicing intermittent fasting, as it can help with weight management, promote blood sugar control, and help maintain muscle mass during weight loss. When practicing intermittent fasting, it is important to be mindful of what you eat during your eating periods, and to prioritize protein, fiber, and healthy fats.

Fats: Its Role in Healthy and Longevity

Fats play an important role in our diet, but not all fats are created equal. Our diets have become inundated with foods full of unhealthy fats and additives, such as saturated and trans fats, that lead to chronic health issues. However, some types of fat are essential for our bodies to function properly and can even aid in improving our health.

Healthy fats, such as monounsaturated and polyunsaturated fats found in avocados, olive oil, nuts, seeds, and fatty fish get lots of focus, but little attention is given to omega-3 EPA (eicosapentaenoic acid) and DHA (docosahexaenoic acid), which are found in some algae, animal foods, and seafood like mackerel, salmon, cod liver, herring, oysters, sardines, anchovies, and caviar. Additionally, omega-6 is found in vegetable oils, nuts, and seeds.

However little attention is given on the significance of having a balanced ratio of omega-3 to omega-6. Excessive intake of omega-6 fatty acids relative to omega-3 fatty acids has been linked to increased inflammation and a risk of chronic diseases such as heart disease and cancer.

When we consume omega-3 and omega-6 in closer to a 1:1 ratio its known to reduce visceral fat by improving metabolic rate, facilitating fat burning, aiding in muscle mass gain, and increasing satiety. It has also shown effectiveness in preventing and managing heart disease, lowering blood pressure, triglycerides, and reducing insulin resistance.[93]

One of the best ways to ensure we are getting the correct amount of healthy fats is through supplementation with omega-3, since getting the right amount of omega-3 from diet alone isn't always easy. Supplementation makes it not only convenient but it's the simplest way to add additional omega-3s to our diet to help you achieve our health goals.

However, not all omega-3 supplements are created equal. It's important to ensure that the source of the omega-3 fish oils is tested for compliance with strict standards for heavy metals like mercury, as well as for appearance, active ingredients, microbial limits, purity, and strength. To learn more about high-quality, concentrated, purified fish oil supplements, visit beyondfeelgreatbook.com.

Micronutrients: Vitamins and Minerals

Micronutrients are nutrients that the body requires for various bodily functions such as metabolism, growth, and development. They are essential to the body, but unlike macronutrients, they are not a significant source of energy. Micronutrients consist of vitamins and minerals, which the body needs in small amounts to function correctly.

Vitamins are organic compounds that play a vital role in various bodily functions, including supporting the immune system, promoting healthy skin, and maintaining vision. They are particularly important in metabolism and include the essential vitamins that the body needs, such as vitamins A, C, D, E, K, and B vitamins such as thiamine (B1), riboflavin (B2), niacin (B3), pantothenic acid (B5), pyroxamine (B6), biotin (B7), folate (B9), and cobalamin (B12). The fat-soluble vitamins A, D, E, and K are stored in the body's fatty tissues and are absorbed best when healthy fats are included in the diet.

Minerals are essential inorganic substances that the body requires for various functions such as building strong bones, regulating fluid balance, and supporting nerve function. Although minerals in foods do not contribute directly to energy needs, they are essential regulators and play a vital role in the body's metabolic pathways. There are more than 50 minerals found in the human body, and about 25 are deemed essential as a deficiency in them can produce specific deficiency symptoms. Important minerals include calcium, phosphorus, iron, sodium, potassium, chloride ions, copper, cobalt, manganese, zinc, magnesium, fluorine, and iodine.

Deficiencies in any of these vitamins and minerals, in and of themselves, could lead to health problems, so it is important to consume a balanced diet that includes a variety of nutrient-dense foods to ensure the body is receiving adequate amounts of essential micronutrients. As we covered throughout this book, the modern dietary intake today is mostly devoid of many of these essential vitamins and minerals. Making supplementation often a necessity. This is why I personally use the *fiber matrix drink,* as it contains a blend of vitamins designed to aid in proper digestion and optimize the conversion of food to fuel.

Digestive Enzymes – "The Workers"

Enzymes and probiotics are important components of a healthy diet that are often overlooked, as they are not classified as macronutrients or micronutrients. Enzymes are the workers in your body that help digest food, regulate organ function, fight viruses and bacteria, and repair cellular damage. They also assist in weight loss by digesting fat. When taken as a supplement with meals, enzymes can break down food in the digestive tract, taking stress off the gallbladder, liver, and pancreas. When taken between meals, they can provide great therapeutic support throughout the entire body.

Enzymes are proteins that facilitate chemical reactions in the body and are essential for various physiological processes, such as digestion, metabolism, and immune system function. There are two types of enzymes: digestive and metabolic enzymes.

Metabolic enzymes are involved in the biochemical reactions that occur in living organisms to sustain life, including the metabolism of various compounds such as carbohydrates, proteins, and fats. They are essential for various biological processes like energy production, cell growth and repair, and waste elimination. Deficiencies in metabolic enzymes can lead to health issues, such as metabolic disorders, digestive problems, and even neurological conditions.[94] Maintaining a healthy balance of metabolic enzymes is crucial for overall health and well-being. This can be achieved by consuming a balanced diet rich in essential macro and micronutrients, ensuring proper digestion, engaging in regular exercise, prioritizing sufficient sleep and stress management, and minimizing exposure to toxins.

Digestive enzymes are secreted along the digestive tract to break food down into nutrients and waste. They are produced mainly by the pancreas, but the liver, gallbladder, small intestine, stomach, and colon also play pivotal roles in their production.[95] Digestive enzymes allow the nutrients in the foods we consume to be absorbed into the bloodstream and the waste to be discarded. The main digestive enzymes made in the pancreas include amylase (breaks down carbohydrates), lipase (breaks down fats), protease (breaks down protein), lactase (breaks down lactose), sucrase (breaks down sucrose) and cellulase (breaks own fiber).

Digestive enzymes are also introduced to the body through raw foods and high-quality supplemental digestion enzyme product, however the body does not produce the enzyme cellulase so it only comes from foods and supplements. However, cooking and processing destroy the enzymes in most of the foods we eat, leaving us with nutrient-poor meals that are harder to digest.

To aid in digestion, it is recommended to use plant-based enzyme supplements that contain they key enzymes like amylase, lipase, protease, and cellulase. Cellulase enzyme is particularly important as the body does not naturally produce it and must rely on external sources such as food or supplements. Digestive enzymes can be taken with meals to ensure efficient food breakdown and absorption, reducing digestive discomforts.[96] They can also provide therapeutic support and contribute to general health and wellness when taken between meals on an empty stomach.

While a healthy diet with raw fruits and vegetables is important, enzyme supplementation, including cellulase, can support optimal health by providing the necessary enzymes for effective food breakdown and nutrient absorption.

Digestive enzyme deficiency can have various implications, including impacts on glucose absorption, weight loss, and insulin resistance. Efficient digestion and breakdown of carbohydrates are vital for proper glucose absorption and utilization.

Insufficient digestive enzymes can hinder carbohydrate breakdown, resulting in impaired glucose absorption, which may contribute to fluctuations in blood sugar levels, difficulties in weight loss, and insulin resistance. Addressing digestive enzyme insufficiency can play a crucial role in optimizing glucose absorption, supporting healthy weight management, and improving insulin sensitivity.

Consider incorporating enzyme supplements into your daily routine for improved digestion and overall wellness. For more information and recommended enzyme supplements that I personally use, visit beyondfeelgreatbook.com.

Probiotics – "Friendly Bacteria"

Enzymes and probiotics play distinct roles in digestion. Probiotics, the beneficial bacteria in your gut, support the work of enzymes by maintaining a healthy digestive tract. However, unlike enzymes, probiotics cannot break down or digest food. Without proper gut bacteria, you may experience symptoms similar to enzyme insufficiency, such as bloating or gas, due to an imbalance in your intestines.

Probiotics are living microorganisms that establish and maintain a healthy balance of beneficial bacteria in the colon and digestive tract, they strengthen the immune system, reduce inflammation, enhance nutrient absorption, contribute to better mental health and prevent harmful bacteria from invading the body. These supplements offer so many health benefits, including addressing gastrointestinal issues like irritable bowel syndrome, Crohn's disease, and food poisoning. They have also been found to prevent vaginal and urinary infections, yeast infections, candida overgrowth, and even reduce the risk of cysts and tumors.[97]

Fermented foods like sauerkraut and a higher fiber dietary intake can also have a significant impact on the gut microbiome.[98] When we consume fiber-rich foods, it passes through the digestive tract largely intact. In the colon, the fiber encounters the gut microbiota, which consists of trillions of bacteria. These bacteria have the ability to break down and ferment certain types of fiber that we cannot digest.[99]

A higher fiber dietary intake promotes the growth of beneficial bacteria in the gut, leading to a more diverse and balanced gut microbiome. This diversity is associated with improved gut health, better digestion, enhanced nutrient absorption, and a reduced risk of certain diseases, including obesity, type 2 diabetes, and cardiovascular disease. For more information on probiotics, visit the resource page at beyondfeelgreatbook.com.

Paving the Way for a Healthier Life

To maintain good health and prevent nutrient deficiencies, consume a balanced diet with a variety of nutrient-dense foods like fruits, vegetables, whole grains, lean proteins, and healthy fats. This helps achieve a balance between carbohydrates, proteins, fats, vitamins, and minerals, supporting overall well-being, immune function, and metabolic health. Incorporating the *fiber matrix drink*, along with digestive enzyme and probiotic supplements, can further serve as important foundations for improved health.

Chapter 11

Active Lifestyle: Anytime, Anywhere

When it comes to leading an active lifestyle, the word "exercise" often conjures up images of sweat-drenched gym equipment or grueling marathon training. However, there's more to fitness than just these traditional forms of exercise. In fact, body weight exercises offer a simple and effective way to improve our health, anytime and anywhere. With body weight exercises, you don't need a gym membership or any equipment - all you need is your own body. By using simple movements, you can challenge your muscles, burn calories, and build strength.

Walking: The Surprising Benefits

Not only is body weight exercise accessible to anyone, it also has many benefits and can be done at any level of health. Walking 30 to 60 minutes a day is highly recommended for individuals seeking to stay fit. Interestingly, a brisk walk has been found to be more effective in maintaining weight than gym exercises or sports.[100] The good news is that walking is a free, fun, and convenient activity that can be easily incorporated into daily routines. All you need is a good pair of shoes and your city's walking trails or sidewalks.

To start, take an easy paced 15-minute walk and gradually increase the time and pace as you build a habit. It's important to keep track of your walks and aim for a brisk pace, where you're breathing noticeably but not out of breath, and can carry on a full conversation while walking. If you have serious health concerns, it's advisable to start at a much slower pace.

The American College of Sports Medicine recommends adding strength training to one's fitness program as it helps burn calories more efficiently, manage chronic conditions, and strengthen bones.[101] While using free weights or weight machines can help you gain strength, body weight exercises have a unique set of benefits, such as building muscle in your core, which can lead to better posture and greater stamina.

Body weight exercises have a lower risk of injury than other exercise techniques. You can easily adjust based on your age, experience, and fitness level, and some body weight exercises are even used to help people recover from injuries. Additionally, body weight exercises can even help your heart. Any kind of exercise is going to help your heart pump blood more effectively, helping you enjoy better circulation and lower blood pressure. But many doctors recommend body weight exercise in particular to patients who are recovering from heart attacks. It's the perfect way to build heart strength and endurance without risking further damage.[102]

Body weight exercises can also improve flexibility. They encourage you to move muscles and joints you may not move otherwise, putting your joints through their full range of movement, which helps them keep moving as they should without risking injury. Strength training and flexibility can easily go hand in hand.

No matter your fitness level, body weight exercise is accessible to anyone. One of the most significant benefits of body weight exercises is that they are free and can be done anywhere, anytime, with no excuses. There are so many different types of movements available that you can easily find a routine that suits your fitness level. By speeding up or slowing down your motion, you can create a more or less challenging workout. You can also choose to do more or fewer repetitions of a given exercise to build a routine best suited to your needs.

You can utilize small pockets of time, such as standing in line, waiting for the microwave, or brushing your teeth, to incorporate exercises into your daily routine. Furthermore, studies have shown that shorter intervals of exercise can be just as beneficial as longer ones, challenging the belief that exercise only counts if you spend at least half an hour at the gym.

Your kitchen, bathroom, or even shower can be perfect places for brief bursts of exercise. You can try counter pushups, coffee stretches and squats, and use your bathroom for exercises like leg lifts or balancing on one foot. Every step counts, and by adding more walking to your day, making exercise a family activity, or finding new ways to challenge yourself, you can keep progressing towards your fitness goals.

Strong Core, Strong Body

The importance of core strength cannot be overstated. If you're looking to lose weight, improve your posture, or have better balance, few things are as effective at achieving these goals as building core strength. Many people associate core exercises with endless series of crunches or sit-ups. While these exercises can help strengthen your abdominals, they are only one part of a healthy core. Your core consists of the muscles in your abdomen, back, and pelvis, which support your spine and help with movement.

Therefore, core strength is crucial for everyone, but it is particularly important for those who suffer from lower back pain. Weak core muscles cannot provide enough support, leading to back pain. Thankfully, prioritizing core strength can help alleviate this pain and prevent future injury.

Your core muscles must work together to help you stay balanced and distribute force evenly, ensuring you exercise safely. If your core muscles are weak, you're more likely to put high levels of stress on other muscles, leading to injury. To keep working towards your goals, it's important to prioritize core strength.

The Benefits of HIIT for Optimal Results

Incorporating high-intensity interval training (HIIT) into your workout routine is an effective way to maximize the benefits of core strength training and improve aerobic and anaerobic fitness, blood pressure, cardiovascular health, insulin sensitivity, cholesterol profiles, and abdominal fat while maintaining muscle mass.[103]

HIIT is a type of exercise that focuses on short bursts of intense activity, followed by longer periods of moderate activity, lasting only a few seconds to a minute. For example, a beginner to HIIT might run as hard as they could for 15 to 30 seconds, then jog or walk for one to two minutes. Alternatively, they may do as many push-ups as they can for 15 seconds, then rest for a minute.

Recent studies have shown that HIIT is one of the most beneficial ways to exercise. This type of training increases your heart rate more efficiently, improves your cardiovascular health, and improves blood flow to the brain, enhancing your thinking and reducing depression.[104] HIIT also increases the use of carbohydrates for energy, reducing insulin levels, both while exercising and for the next 24 to 48 hours. You don't need any equipment to do HIIT; you can exercise in intervals using only your body weight, anywhere, anytime. It burns calories efficiently, helping you lose more weight in less time.

The benefits of HIIT are not limited to just burning calories. A 2011 paper published in the Journal of Obesity highlighted the numerous benefits of high-intensity exercise, suggesting that HIIT may be more effective at reducing abdominal fat and cellulite than any other type of exercise.[105] The research also suggested that HIIT not only helps your body burn calories while active but also increases calorie burning while at rest, even hours after exercising.

By limiting yourself to just 20 minutes of high-intensity interval training and incorporating it into your routine, you can achieve your fitness goals quickly and efficiently. By building core strength and using HIIT, you'll look better, feel better, and be able to carry out everyday tasks more easily.

In conclusion, it is important to make exercise a consistent part of your daily routine in order to achieve your fitness goals, whether you are trying to lose weight, build muscle, or improve your overall health. It is important to remember that reaching your health goals is a journey, not a destination, and requires time, effort, dedication, and consistency to see results. By incorporating body weight exercises into your routine and making exercise a habit, you can improve your overall health and well-being for years to come.

Chapter 12

Healthy Habits: For Lifelong Success

Prioritizing healthy habits is critical to achieving positive change in our overall health. By focusing on habit stacking, we can set ourselves up for a healthier and happier future without making all the changes at once. While developing healthy habits can be challenging, making them a priority can improve our quality of life and help us live our best life.

In this chapter, we will explore ten key habits for a healthy life. Building healthy habits requires a shift in mindset and a willingness to make sacrifices to improve our health. Regardless of age, gender, or physical ability, investing in healthy habits is a worthy investment in our health and well-being.

To begin building healthy habits, it's essential to understand the role they play in our daily routines. Habits are small, automatic actions that we do without much thought, such as brushing our teeth in the morning or taking a walk after dinner. They become powerful because they require minimal effort or motivation once formed and become a natural part of our daily routine.

The first step towards a healthier life is committing to building healthy habits. Rather than relying on quick fixes or temporary changes, we must make healthy habits a permanent lifestyle change to achieve long-term success in improving our health and well-being. By incorporating healthy habits into our daily routines, we can achieve lifelong success in our journey towards optimal health.

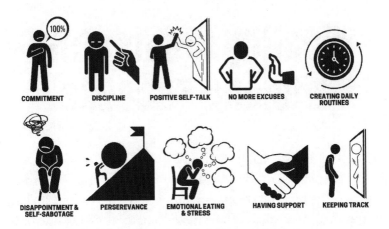

COMMITMENT   DISCIPLINE   POSITIVE SELF-TALK   NO MORE EXCUSES   CREATING DAILY ROUTINES

DISAPPOINTMENT & SELF-SABOTAGE   PERSEREVANCE   EMOTIONAL EATING & STRESS   HAVING SUPPORT   KEEPING TRACK

Staying Committed: Navigating the Ups and Downs

The good news is that building healthy habits is not as difficult as you might think. With a little bit of effort and commitment, anyone can start building healthy habits that will last a lifetime. Whether you're looking to control blood sugars, lose weight, get more exercise, or eat healthier, the principles for building healthy habits are the same. By taking small, consistent actions each day, you can make healthy habits a natural part of your life. So, let's dive in and start building those healthy habits for life!

As you embark on the journey of building healthy habits, you will undoubtedly encounter distractions that threaten to derail your progress. With a busy schedule and countless demands on your time, it can be all too easy to let healthy habits fall by the wayside. That's why it's important to have a plan in place to keep distractions at bay.

One way to minimize distractions is to remove them from your environment. Block out time in your schedule each day to prioritize physical activity, clear your cupboards of unhealthy foods that may tempt you, and get rid of any other distractions that could pull you away from your goals.

Another roadblock that may arise is a lack of discipline. It's natural to have days when you don't feel like exercising or sticking to a healthy eating plan. But discipline is what will keep you on track, even when motivation is low. As you progress through the challenge, you will have the opportunity to develop your discipline skills and become even more committed to your healthy habits.

Finally, the fear of leaving your comfort zone can be a significant obstacle to building healthy habits. Making changes to your dietary lifestyle can be challenging and unfamiliar, and it's normal to feel a little nervous about stepping outside your comfort zone. But don't let fear hold you back from following through on the commitment you've made to yourself. Embrace the discomfort and take each day as an opportunity to learn and grow. With commitment, discipline, and a willingness to step outside your comfort zone, you can build healthy habits that will last a lifetime.

The Power of Discipline: Unlocking Success

Discipline is a critical ingredient in achieving success in all aspects of life, including personal, professional, and health-related goals. When you have discipline, you can stay focused and committed to your objectives, even when it's difficult, and resist the temptation to be sidetracked by distractions or setbacks.

The lack of discipline can hinder your progress and prevent you from achieving your goals. You may find it challenging to stay motivated, give in to short-term pleasures, and struggle to maintain a healthy balance between work and rest. Procrastination, negative habits, and impulsive behavior can also interfere with your ability to stay on track.

Research has demonstrated that discipline is a more significant factor in long-term success than intelligence or talent. If you want to make positive changes in your life and achieve your goals, developing discipline is vital.

Building discipline can be challenging, but it's worth the effort. A great place to start is by removing distractions, temptations, or negative influences from your environment. Establishing a consistent routine, such as going to bed and waking up at the same time every day, can also create structure and enhance productivity.

It is also important to tune out naysayers and focus on your own path, rather than getting discouraged by negative comments from others. Tracking your progress is another effective method to stay motivated and celebrate your accomplishments. Recognize that every small step towards your goal is a result of discipline and self-control.

As you continue to practice discipline, you will find it becomes more comfortable to make the right choices, and you'll stay more focused and motivated. With discipline and commitment, you can make positive changes in your life and achieve your goals.

The Power of Self-Talk: Your Thoughts

The person you speak to the most throughout the day isn't your spouse, your children, or your coworkers - it's yourself. The way you talk to yourself can have a significant impact on your thoughts, actions, and accomplishments. That's why keeping a positive attitude and being mindful of the messages you give yourself is crucial to reaching your goals.

When you maintain a positive attitude towards yourself and your goals, you're less likely to feel stressed. Having a positive outlook helps you manage stress better, leading to improved health and faster goal attainment. When you practice positive self-talk, you feel better about yourself, appreciate the good things in your life, focus on your strengths, and feel motivated to overcome obstacles. This, in turn, leads to a more fulfilling life and better stress management. On the other hand, negative self-talk can lead to feeling worse about yourself, constantly focusing on what you lack, underestimating your abilities, and struggling to find motivation to push through obstacles. Negative self-talk can lead to an unhappy, unproductive, and unfulfilling life, and have a negative impact on your stress management.

You might think that ideas such as positivity and kindness to oneself are just nice things to hear, but research shows they have scientific merit. For example, a 2011 study by a psychology researcher at the University of North Carolina found that a meditation practice aimed at improving positivity and self-talk, had a profound effect on participants.[106] Compared to the control group, the meditation group had a greater sense of purpose in life, better relationships, and fewer symptoms of illness. These positive changes are linked to a more fulfilling life and reduced risk of depression. In other words, being kind to yourself and practicing positivity lead to a healthier, happier, and more fulfilling life.

Aside from helping you maintain a positive attitude, being mindful of your self-talk is also crucial for managing stress. Unchecked stress can have a detrimental impact on your health and well-being, as it is known to trigger physical symptoms such as high blood pressure and cardiovascular issues; as well as lead to weight gain and unhealthy food choices. Negative self-talk can worsen the effects of stress, leading to a downward spiral that takes a toll on your quality of life.

The good news is that you have the power to control your thoughts and shift from negative to positive self-talk. Start by paying attention to the messages you give yourself and try to replace negative thoughts with positive ones. You can also try mindfulness meditation, which is scientifically proven to reduce stress and have a positive impact on your body. Writing your thoughts down in a journal and identifying consistent stressors in your life can also help you reduce anxious feelings. Remember to forgive yourself for past mistakes, practice gratitude by acknowledging the good things in your life, and seek out positive people and experiences.

With practice, positivity and self-kindness can become natural; leading to a happier, healthier, and more fulfilling life.

Recognizing Excuses: Roadblocks to Success

Excuses can be the biggest roadblocks to achieving our goals. Whether it's lack of time, age, or other circumstances, the more we rely on excuses, the further we will be from our objectives. It is crucial to recognize that excuses not only hinder our progress, but also affect our attitudes towards ourselves and our world.

When we make excuses for not taking care of our bodies, eating well, or performing at work, we prevent ourselves from reaching our full potential. Excuses also create a vicious cycle of negative self-talk, self-doubt, and victimhood, leading to feelings of worthlessness and depression. Overcoming the habit of excuses is crucial for long-term health and wellness.

To take responsibility for our lives, we must stop relying on excuses and shift our mindset. If we're not where we want to be, we can still achieve new goals, but we must make changes to get different results. Excuses are a convenient way to avoid accountability, but they ultimately lead us to abandon our goals and settle for less.

To avoid falling into the trap of excuses, surround yourself with positive and inspiring people who are in the same journey as you. Being around people who make excuses can be contagious and hold you back from reaching your potential. When old excuses try to creep back into your life, don't beat yourself up over them.

Instead, address them head-on, reset your thinking, and keep moving forward towards your goals.

Building Healthy Habits: Establishing Routines

In our fast-paced lives, we're constantly faced with numerous small decisions that can quickly become overwhelming. Often, the busyness and chaos can cause important areas such as exercise, eating right, and sleep, to fall by the wayside. This can have a negative impact on our health, weight, and overall wellness. However, there is a solution - creating daily routines.

By establishing routines, we can ensure that the most important things get done, and take some of the stress from planning our day, allowing us to focus on more important tasks. Everyone has activities they enjoy and those they don't, as well as tasks that require immediate attention and those that can be put off, such as exercising or getting enough sleep. With so much to accomplish daily, creating routines can free up our time and energy by eliminating the need to constantly make decisions about what to do next.

One of the significant benefits of routines is they allow us to make decisions in advance, taking the guesswork out of our daily schedules. For instance, if we establish a routine of visiting the gym before work, we've already decided to do so. Similarly, if we create a habit of preparing a healthy meal and going to bed at a regular time, we're much more likely to follow through. The decision has already been made, eliminating the need to constantly evaluate our choices.

Another advantage of routines is that, with time, they become automatic and save us time. To start creating routines, identify three areas of your life that would benefit from having daily routines, such as your eating habits, exercise routine, sleep schedule, or stress management techniques. By creating and sticking to these routines, you will ensure that these areas remain a priority, leading to a healthier, happier life.

Initially, establishing routines might require some effort and discipline, and it may take some time for them to become automatic. However, over time, they will become more and more natural, allowing you to make healthy decisions without a second thought.

Creating and sticking to routines can make a significant difference in our weight, body, and life. Are you ready to commit to establishing and maintaining routines to achieve your goals and improve your overall well-being?

The Internal Struggle: Recognizing Self-Sabotage

Working towards your goals can be challenging, especially when you don't receive the support you need from those around you. This is particularly true when they actively work against you or express their opposition to your goals. However, it is not just external factors that can sabotage your progress - sometimes we're our own worst enemy. So, let's review the causes and effects of self-sabotage, as well as practical tips to overcome it and achieve your goals.

The people you surround yourself with can play a significant role in your health and weight loss journey. A study conducted in 2014 followed a group of women who were trying to lose weight over a period of a year and half. They were asked to keep track of the feedback they received from others about their weight. Those who reported receiving more positive feedback were able to maintain their weight loss long after the study ended, and those who received fewer positive messages were unsuccessful at maintaining it after the program ended.[107]

Your loved ones may try to sabotage your efforts for various reasons. Perhaps they're envious of your progress, worried that you will leave them behind if you make changes, or simply want to control your life. Whatever the reason, their behavior can slow you down or even cause you to give up altogether.

So, how do you spot a saboteur? Look out for people who exhibit the following behaviors: The Envious One: someone who seems happy for your weight loss success, but is actually envious and resentful. They may make subtle digs or detract from your achievements.

It is also important to monitor any self-sabotaging behavior. Pay attention to what you think or say to yourself when you engage in such behavior. Write down your thoughts, even if they seem silly or unrealistic. Then, challenge these thoughts by asking yourself questions. Why are you behaving in a way that keeps you from achieving your goals? What beliefs are guiding your self-sabotage? Are these beliefs based on facts or past failures that prevent you from moving forward?

To combat self-sabotage, develop thoughts and behaviors that support your goals. When you find yourself engaging in self-sabotaging thoughts, encourage and motivate yourself. Focus on your past successes, and build self-confidence. It's important to be patient and persistent, as it may take time to turn a saboteur into a supporter. If someone you love is resistant to your lifestyle changes, don't let their negativity hold you back. Keep working on your goals and be an example of what's possible when you commit to making positive changes in your life.

Developing a Persevering Mindset

Achieving long-lasting change in your life can be a difficult and challenging journey. You may work hard for weeks, months, or even years, but all your progress can be undone if you slip back into old habits. The good news is there is a cure for this: perseverance.

When you commit to persevering through tough times, working towards your goals, and refusing to let little issues throw you off track, you can make lasting change. Over the course of your challenge, you have worked on creating change in many areas of your life, but the most important change you can make is the decision to persevere. By committing to perseverance, you ensure that the changes you have made will stick.

Approaching your goals with a persevering mindset means having a long-term perspective that encourages patience, short-term sacrifice, and the ability to move past failures quickly. By doing so, you can achieve your goals, lose more weight, and experience changes that last. However, if you overlook the importance of perseverance, setbacks and failures can derail your progress, and you may even start to gain weight again.

Perseverance is especially crucial in weight loss. A 2016 study from the University of Copenhagen found that people who persevered in their weight loss plan were more likely to keep it off.[108] These individuals experienced changes in their hunger-related hormone levels, with lower levels of the hormone that causes a large appetite and higher levels of the hormone that helps them feel full. By persevering through obstacles and sticking to your plan, you are more likely to reach and maintain your goal weight.

To develop a persevering mindset, recognize that it's a skill you can grow and develop, rather than an innate personality trait. Listen to the little voice in your head that tells you to stay in your comfort zone, and challenge negative thoughts that may lead you astray. Keep your eyes on the goal; set specific and achievable goals, and establish deadlines to keep your enthusiasm up. When you're tempted to give up, promise yourself you will do just one more thing.

To maintain your perseverance skills over the long term, take care of yourself by getting enough rest, managing stress, and eating healthy. Surround yourself with a supportive community, and take responsibility for your actions and mistakes to avoid blaming others. By building up your perseverance skills, you will ensure that you continue to work towards your goals, even in the face of obstacles.

Emotional Triggers: Unhealthy Eating

Emotional eating is a common cause of weight gain, where people use food as a way to cope with their emotions instead of satisfying hunger. If you are trying to lose weight, improve your diet, and lead a healthier lifestyle, it is important to recognize the connection between your emotions and your eating habits.

Many of us may not realize we turn to food to deal with our feelings. However, understanding what triggers emotional eating can help us change this behavior. Whether it's reaching for a pint of ice cream after a breakup, snacking while working on a stressful project, or eating just because we're bored, emotional eating can have negative effects on our weight, health, and wellbeing.

It is important to recognize that emotional eating is not just associated with negative emotions. Some people indulge in food as a reward when they're happy or celebrating. For others, eating a large portion of a favorite recipe may provide comfort. Regardless of the reason, emotional eating can have consequences, so it is important to learn how to unlearn these patterns and replace them with healthier ones.

A 2012 study found that people who learned to regulate their emotions instead of suppressing them were less likely to turn to food as a way to cope with negative experiences.[109]

If you find yourself eating in response to emotions, it is essential to rethink your response. Next time you feel the urge to eat for emotional reasons, hit the pause button. Ask yourself questions such as what you're feeling and whether you're actually really hungry. Weigh the consequences and choose a smarter solution. Replace old patterns of emotional eating with healthier habits.

Emotional eating can hinder your progress in reaching your goals. To change your relationship with food, try being more conscious of why you're eating. Before you eat, go through the three steps of thinking, weighing, and acting, to ensure you are eating for the right reasons. With practice, you can avoid emotional eating altogether and enjoy a healthier lifestyle.

Eliminating emotional eating is an important part of leading a healthy lifestyle in the long term. You can practice mindful eating by paying close attention to, and fully experiencing the foods you eat. Track the physical sensations you experience to distinguish emotional cravings from true hunger. Enjoy your favorite foods in moderation, like treating yourself to a small piece of chocolate once a week, and forgive yourself for slip-ups. Learn from your experiences and move on with your healthy habits.

Having a Champion for Support

Making significant lifestyle changes, such as eating healthier and exercising, is a challenging process that requires time and hard work. While many people may overlook the importance of support, it can be more critical to success than they realize. A champion for support consists of individuals who are aware of the healthy lifestyle changes you are making, and are committed to supporting you through the process. This can include almost anyone, from your significant other, family members, friends, business associates and coworkers.

Those you live with and spend the most time with are the most important champions to support you. It is critical that you discuss your goals and plan lifestyle changes with your significant other, spouse, family, and children, and ask for their unwavering support. By promoting a healthy lifestyle through your example, you can help them create habits that will serve them for the rest of their life.

Sharing your planned lifestyle changes and motivation with your champion is essential to increase your chances of making healthy lifestyle changes and maintaining them long term. The resulting support from loved ones, as well as an added measure of accountability, is imperative when making a permanent lifestyle change.

Your champion can provide accountability, encouragement, and positivity in various ways. For example, you might start an accountability text, or ask someone to be your exercise partner. You can also benefit from emotional, nutritional, exercise, and inspirational support.

Your champion can be crucial to creating a healthy new lifestyle, so don't underestimate the power of surrounding yourself with positive and supportive people. Making lifestyle changes can be challenging, and you want to be with people who will give you the very best chance of success.

The Importance of Keeping Track

At the start of your journey towards a healthier lifestyle, it is important to begin documenting your progress. Tracking your progress is essential for achieving your goals and maintaining your momentum for the long term. It is such a vital part of your experience.

Measuring your progress and taking regular measurements is a critical aspect of achieving any goal. Imagine if baseball players didn't know their batting averages, or if students didn't receive their test scores. How would they know if they were improving or if their hard work was paying off? In short, what you measure, you can achieve.

Simply having something measured motivates us to work harder and perform better. This is true whether it's in school, at work, in competition, or when making lifestyle changes.

When you track and measure your progress, you can set your goals more effectively. You can evaluate your progress intelligently, understand where you stand, identify areas for improvement, and troubleshoot any issues that are holding you back. Most importantly, by tracking progress at the beginning of your journey, you will be able to look back and see how far you've come.

Measuring your progress is essential for staying motivated and reaching your goals. Take your initial measurements today and let your challenge team know that you've started. Then, look forward to the change you will see once you have completed this challenge. When you look back over your progress, you will have plenty to celebrate.

In this chapter, we've discussed several approaches to developing and maintaining healthy habits, with a particular emphasis on two strategies: habit stacking and gradual habit formation. Habit stacking involves linking new habits to existing ones, which makes it easier to adopt them as part of your daily routine.

Gradual habit formation, on the other hand, is just starting with one habit and building up to multiple healthy habits over time. For example, you could begin by exercising for just 10 minutes a day and gradually increase the frequency or duration of your workouts time. By combining these approaches, you can establish healthy habits that are simpler to maintain and that promote a healthier and more fulfilling life.

Chapter 13

— *ell* —

Supplements: Worth The Hype or Help?

As the number of health-conscious consumers grows, the health and wellness industry is experiencing a significant boom. This has led to an abundance of supplements, healthy branded foods, and various products that claim to promote optimal health and well-being. However, it is essential to be aware that not all marketers are sincere in their promotions, and there can be considerable differences in the quality and safety of products. Consequently, consumers must exercise diligence in researching and choosing products to make informed decisions for their overall health and well-being.

Nutrient Content: Challenges for a Healthier Diet

In recent years, there has been growing concern about the nutritional value of the food we eat. While fruits and vegetables are still widely regarded as healthy, nutrient-rich foods, many people are discovering that eating a diet rich in these foods does not necessarily mean they are getting all the nutrition they need.

Research indicates that the nutrient content of the foods we eat has declined over the years. A 2004 study published in the Journal of the American College of Nutrition found that the amount of six important nutrients - protein, calcium, phosphorus, iron, vitamin B2, and vitamin C - declined in 43 foods from 1950 to 1999.[110]

The result of this trend is that millions of people are lacking the basic building blocks necessary for a healthy body.

One reason for the decline in nutrient content is the pressure to produce more food from the same land. With the population growing exponentially, there is simply not enough land to produce food for everyone without sacrificing nutritional content. This has resulted in a decline in soil quality, which leads to a decrease in the nutritional value of the food we eat.

Another reason for the decline in nutrient content is the rise of processed, factory-made ultra-processed foods. These foods do not contain the nutrients necessary for a healthy diet. Our ancestors, who lived on wild foods, consumed high levels of essential fats, minerals, and vitamins, whereas today's foods do not compare. Additionally, environmental toxins, lack of sunlight, and chronic stress increase our need for nutrients.

Supplements: Filling Nutritional Gaps

Evidence now suggests that certain supplements are essential and can support health in a variety of ways, but not all supplements are created equal.[111] And with how busy and hectic life can get, taking the time to sit down and eat all the required nutrients is both unrealistic and near impossible, considering the nutrient value of foods today. Supplements can support any on-the-go, quick-paced lifestyle so you don't have to compromise your nutrient intake. Supplements can offer the nutrients we wouldn't otherwise receive.

Other medical conditions make supplements a necessity. For example, adults diagnosed with osteoporosis require extra vitamin D in addition to what they get from their regular diets, and those who are diabetic, the *fiber matrix drink* can slow down the absorption of sugar in the body, helping to control blood sugar levels. Additionally, fiber supplements can reduce cholesterol, blood sugar, and triglycerides without requiring dangerous drugs or drastic dietary changes. If you're interested in these benefits, the *fiber matrix drink* may be suitable for you. To learn more about the *fiber matrix drink* I recommend, visit beyondfeelgreatbook.com.

While supplements can be beneficial and effective, it's important to remember they should not just replace a healthy dietary lifestyle. Supplements are designed to supplement a healthy lifestyle; they do not create it. Supplements provide a way to fill the gaps in our diets caused by nutrient depletion, processed foods, and other factors.

Dietary supplements have gained increasing consumer interest in recent years, and they are only continuing to rise in popularity. The supplement industry is a billion-dollar market, and it's no surprise that many companies are looking to cash in on the trend. A 2019 market analysis showed that the global dietary supplement market is expected to reach 216.3 billion in USD, by 2026.[112] With that statistic, and over 90,000 vitamin varieties available, it's clear that supplements play an important part in nutrition.

Navigating the Supplement Industry

Despite the popularity of supplements, it's important to ask whether they truly live up to their claims of improving our health. As consumers, it's important to be aware of the reality of the supplement industry. We should always do our research when choosing which supplements to take. One example is the multivitamin, an iconic and best-selling supplement that has been around since 1936 when it was first developed in Switzerland. Despite its popularity, recent research suggests that the standard multivitamin may not be effective in maintaining human health, particularly given current lifestyle and dietary factors.

Consumers typically make buying decisions when purchasing nutritional supplements based on a variety of factors, such as their personal health needs, recommendations from others, marketing claims, availability and accessibility of the product, and price. It is important to prioritize quality, as well-made, science-based supplements are almost always a better choice than the sugary vitamin gummies found at local drugstores.

One of the most important factors to consider when purchasing supplements is transparency. When it comes to transparency, there are a few key areas to consider. First, it's important to know who the actual manufacturer is of the supplement. As consumers, it's hard to know who the actual manufacturer is and what science, if any, is behind the product formulas. The truth is that while there are thousands of brands and varieties, there are actually a small number of manufacturers.

Thanks to technology and efficient supply chains, anyone can now enter the supplement market and become their own supplement brand for a small investment. I recently saw an ad on social media promoting that anyone can now start their own supplements line 'for as little as $197'. The company's claim is that they purchase in bulk quantities from the supplement manufacturers, warehouse the inventory, and simply add a private label for you to sell to consumers. The reality of the supplement industry is that, for most retailers, the only difference from one bottle to the next is the private labelling, and sometimes a slight variation in the formula.

Another important aspect of transparency is the science behind the products. Many companies, in their marketing and promotions, make claims about the benefits of their products without providing any scientific evidence to back up those claims. It's important to look for companies who have a strong commitment to research and development and who provide access to scientific studies and clinical trials that support their products.

Finally, transparency also extends to the supply chain and manufacturing process. As consumers, we want to know where the raw materials are sourced and how the products are produced. Are they produced in a GMP certified facility? Are they tested for purity and potency?

Choosing Quality Supplements: Transparency

A supplement company must be committed to full transparency and ownership of their products, from the science and research to the sourcing, manufacturing, distribution, and delivery. Do they have their own FDA approved (or a similar standard in your country) manufacturing facilities, ensuring the highest quality and purity? Do they conduct extensive testing for all their raw ingredients to ensure the purity and potency are consistent? Do they employ a dedicated team of scientists and researchers who work to develop products that are backed by science and clinical trials?

I've conducted my own thorough research, and personally only use and recommend supplements from companies who are the actual manufacturers and have transparency. If you're interested in the supplements I take and endorse, which meet these specific criteria, I invite you to visit beyondfeelgreatbook.com. On the website, you'll find links where I explain in detail the distinguishing factors of these supplements compared to others in the global industry.

The products that have made the biggest difference in my health are the *fiber matrix drink* and *yerba mate drink*, mentioned in this book. The *fiber matrix drink* consists of a unique combination of soluble and insoluble fibers that support healthy digestion and maintain healthy blood sugar levels. The *yerba mate drink* is an energizing beverage with antioxidants and other beneficial nutrients. It can prolong fasting periods by curbing hunger, boosting energy levels, enhancing mental clarity, and fostering a sense of well-being. Additionally, it serves as a great alternative to coffee or sugary energy drinks.

After conducting thorough research, I've found that what sets these products apart from other supplement providers is the manufacturer's unwavering commitment to quality, safety, and transparency. They use only the finest ingredients, and take a comprehensive approach to scientific research, clinical studies, and quality assurance - from farming and cultivating raw materials on their own land resources throughout the world, to the development process.

In a recent study, the scientists looked at how the daily use of the *fiber matrix drink* as well as the *yerba mate drink* during a period of intermittent fasting, affected the cardiometabolic health of healthy adults. Participants fasted overnight for 14-16 hours each day. Measurements were taken at the beginning, middle, and end of the 60-day study period to track changes in weight, waist circumference, blood lipids, and glycated hemoglobin (HbA1c) levels.[113]

The results showed that participants experienced significant improvements in their cardiometabolic health, including lower levels of non-HDL, LDL, and total cholesterol, as well as lower triglyceride and HbA1c levels. There were also significant decreases in body weight and waist circumference. The study found that the combination of this system had a greater impact on those with higher starting levels of non-HDL cholesterol. Their conclusion was that this system improved important markers of cardiovascular and metabolic health in healthy adults over a 60-day period and it is an effective way to improve cardiometabolic health outcomes. For the study results visit beyondfeelgreatbook.com to download document.

Understanding the realities of the supplement industry and conducting thorough research when selecting products is crucial for consumers. This ensures that you choose top-quality, food-based supplements sourced directly from a reputable, science-based manufacturer, rather than from an obscure marketing company that merely puts a private label on the packaging. It's important to prioritize quality over quantity when selecting supplements.

In addition to the criteria mentioned earlier, there are a few more things to consider when purchasing nutritional supplements. Firstly, look for supplements that are third-party tested for purity and potency, which can ensure that the supplement contains the ingredients listed on the label and in the correct amounts, and that it is free from contaminants. Secondly, check the ingredient list for any potential allergens or intolerances. Thirdly, consider the form of the supplement, such as capsules, tablets, liquid or powdered form. Fourthly, check the dosage instructions and follow them carefully. Finally, be cautious of supplement marketeers who make exaggerated or unsupported claims.

By selecting high-quality supplements that meet all of these criteria, consumers can feel confident that they are treating their body to only the best nutritional supplements and getting the best value for their health.

Chapter 14

Common Mistakes: Avoiding Obstacles

In the pursuit of better health and weight loss, it's easy to fall into the trap of making common mistakes. From low calorie diets to keto and low fat diets, there are countless approaches to glucose control and weight loss, each with its own set of potential pitfalls. Not eating enough protein, only focusing on the scale, snacking, and not tracking foods are just a few of the missteps that can sabotage progress.

The challenges of eating out too often, inadequate sleep, high stress levels, and insufficient meal planning can make it difficult to stick to a healthy routine. It's important to understand these common mistakes and how to avoid them in order to achieve your health and weight loss goals. By paying attention to key factors such as protein intake, water consumption, and alcohol consumption, as well as seeking out support and developing a solid meal planning strategy, you can set yourself up for success on your weight loss journey.

By the end of this chapter, you'll have a better understanding of these common mistakes and how to avoid them, giving you the tools you need to succeed in your health and weight loss journey.

The Impact of Low-Calorie Diets

A low-calorie diet can cause a decrease in the hormone leptin, which regulates your metabolism. This can make your body believe it's starving, leading to a downgrade of your thyroid and a lower metabolic rate. As a result, any incoming calories may be stored as fat since your body isn't able to sustain the low-calorie diet.

Additionally, when combined with increased physical activity, low-calorie diets can raise the hormone cortisol, leading to the breakdown of lean muscle mass. Although you may initially see weight loss results on the scale, the unsustainable approach can sacrifice optimal metabolic health and turn your body into a fat-storing machine rather than a fat-burning one. It's important to remember that muscle weighs more than fat.

Not Eating Enough Protein

Adequate protein consumption is crucial for glucose control and weight loss. It offers various benefits such as reducing appetite, protecting muscle mass, increasing satiety, and improving metabolic rate. Despite its vital importance as a foundational nutrient, protein is often overlooked, as discussed in Chapter 10.

Beyond the Scale: Measuring Progress

Relying solely on the scale to measure weight loss progress can be misleading as weight can fluctuate daily due to various factors such as fluid retention, undigested food, and bowel movements. To accurately track progress, it is recommended to take measurements of your waist and to use before pictures as a reference. Additionally, it is important to pay attention to how you feel, your blood sugar and energy levels throughout the day, and how you are sleeping as these factors can be key indicators of progress. By looking beyond the scale and considering multiple measures of progress, you can better track your weight loss journey and stay motivated to reach your goals.

Consuming Processed "Diet" Foods

Processed "diet" foods, including low-fat, keto, and other similar products, can be tempting when trying to lose weight. However, these processed food items are often filled with unknown ingredients and are made in factories, coming in boxes, bags, and labeled with bar codes.

Despite being marketed as low-fat, low-calorie, or keto-friendly, these foods often contain high amounts of unwanted ingredients that can promote insulin resistance and hinder weight loss progress.

To optimize your health and weight loss goals, it is best to make every effort to stay away from processed foods and focus on whole, nutrient-dense foods that are fresh and minimally processed. By avoiding the dangers of processed "diet" foods, you can achieve sustainable weight loss and improve your overall health and well-being.

Re-evaluate Snacking Habits

Snacking can be a common pitfall when trying to achieve sustainable weight loss. If you find yourself constantly snacking throughout the day, it may be beneficial to take a closer look at what you're eating during meals. Ensure that you're consuming enough protein and be aware of snacking as an emotional attachment or habit.

Incorporating an intermittent fasting routine, concentrated yerba mate drink in the morning, and a fiber matrix drink before meals can help achieve better long-term weight loss results. Intermittent fasting can help reduce the urge to snack and improve insulin sensitivity, while yerba mate and fiber matrix drinks can help promote satiety and support healthy digestion.

By re-evaluating your snacking habits and incorporating these strategies, you can achieve sustainable weight loss and improve your overall health and well-being.

Food Tracking for Success

Not tracking the foods you consume can be a common mistake when starting a weight loss journey. Tracking what you eat can help you better understand the types and amounts of nutrients you are consuming and how they impact your weight loss progress.

Studies have shown that food tracking can improve self-accountability and help provide a better understanding of the amounts of macronutrients consumed on a daily basis. By keeping track of your food intake, you can identify patterns and adjust your diet to better support your weight loss goals.

At the beginning of your weight loss journey, it can be particularly beneficial to track your food intake. This can help you establish healthy habits and support long-term success. With the help of food tracking, you can achieve sustainable weight loss and improve your overall health and well-being.

The Power of Community Support

Embarking on a weight loss journey alone can be challenging and can significantly reduce the chances of success. Studies have shown that trying to lose weight alone can result in a lower success rate however; by joining a community of individuals with similar health goals for support, can mean the difference between success and failure.[114]

Having a community to hold you accountable, encourage you, and provide support can make all the difference in achieving your weight loss goals. When you are feeling down or discouraged, your community can provide you with the confidence and motivation to keep pushing forward towards success.

By not having support, you risk missing out on a powerful resource that can help you achieve sustainable weight loss and improve your overall health and well-being. Joining a community of like-minded individuals can help keep you accountable and motivated, making your weight loss journey both enjoyable and successful.

Eating Out Too Often

Eating out frequently can be a common pitfall when trying to achieve sustainable weight loss. Restaurants often prioritize taste, texture, and flavor over health, leading to menus filled with sugar-laden and inflammatory oil-cooked fast foods served in larger than normal portions. In addition, indulging in drinks and side dishes that one would not normally consume at home can lead to excess calorie intake.

Eating out too often can also make it challenging to track the types and amounts of nutrients consumed, making it difficult to stay within your daily calorie limit. By opting to cook at home more often, you can control the ingredients and portion sizes of your meals and make healthier choices that support your weight loss goals.

It's important to be mindful of the risks of eating out too often and make conscious efforts to limit restaurant meals. By incorporating healthy meal planning and cooking at home, you can achieve sustainable weight loss and improve your overall health and well-being.

The Impact of Sleep and Stress

When it comes to weight loss, it's not just about diet and exercise. Sleep and stress also play a significant role in your progress.

Research has shown that lack of sleep and high stress levels can contribute to weight gain and difficulty losing weight.

Getting enough sleep is essential for maintaining optimal health and supporting weight loss. Lack of sleep can lead to hormonal imbalances, which can directly impact weight loss or gain. In addition, stress can increase cortisol levels, which often results in overeating or poor food choices.

Studies have found that the amount of sleep you get and your body's ability to manage weight and blood sugar are closely connected. For example, a University of Chicago study found that when two groups of people ate the same number of calories, the group that got only five and a half hours of sleep per night lost about six and a half pounds less than the people who had a full eight and a half hours of sleep.[115]

To support better sleep and lower stress levels, it's important to establish healthy habits and routines. This can include setting a sleep schedule and sticking to it, creating a relaxing bedtime ritual, and making your bedroom sleep-friendly by adjusting the temperature, reducing noise, and minimizing light.

It's also important to avoid consuming caffeine, alcohol, or nicotine in the afternoon or evening, as well as having overly large meals close to bedtime. Physical activity throughout the day can help you fall asleep and stay asleep, but be cautious of exercising too close to bedtime.

By making these changes and prioritizing sleep and stress management, you can support your weight loss journey and overall health and well-being.

Portion Control and Meal Planning

Proper nutrition is crucial for a healthy body. While exercise is important, 80% of weight loss results come from your diet. To improve your metabolism and lose weight, it's essential to consider the size and content of your meals. Meal planning and portion control can help you make small yet significant changes to your eating habits.

By planning your meals and controlling portions, you consume fewer calories, which helps with weight loss and blood sugar control. A healthy balanced diet includes reasonable portion sizes, whole grains, lean cuts of meat, fish, fruits, vegetables, legumes, healthy fats, and dairy. Avoid foods high in saturated and trans fats, high glycemic snacks, and sugary desserts.

Read food labels to determine which foods to include in your diet and how much to eat. Look for foods high in fiber, healthy fats, and protein. Pay attention to serving sizes as they may be smaller than you think.

Use the plate method to portion out your meals. Divide a nine-inch dinner plate in half and divide one of the halves again. The largest section should be filled with non-starchy vegetables, while the smaller section should contain healthy carbohydrates and lean protein. You may also include a serving of dairy, fruit, or healthy fat, as long as it doesn't exceed your caloric goals.

Be flexible with your meal planning. If the plate method doesn't work for you, try counting carbohydrates or tracking calories. Don't give up if a particular method doesn't work. Making small, sustainable changes to your diet is key to long-term success.

Water and Hydration

Did you know that your body is 60% water? If you're not regularly rehydrating, your health may be at risk. Drinking water not only keeps you healthy, but it's also scientifically proven to help you lose weight. If weight loss is your goal, drinking water is essential to getting there. In fact, getting enough sleep is just as important as staying hydrated when it comes to losing weight, being healthy, and living your best life.

When you drink enough water, you can enjoy many benefits, including consuming fewer calories from liquids, replenishing water lost during exercise, removing toxins that can cause skin issues, boosting energy levels, reducing digestion problems, and refreshing your mood. On the other hand, failing to drink enough water can lead to weight gain from drinking liquid carbohydrates, dry skin, sleepiness, more headaches, difficulty concentrating, and increased appetite due to feeling less full.

Drinking water is not only necessary for staying healthy; it can also help increase weight loss. A 2007 study found that low drinking water intake was associated with various unhealthful behaviors, including low levels of physical activity and low levels of fruit and vegetable intake.[116] If you're struggling to cut back on your food intake, drinking water can help you feel full and make it easier to reduce calories. Additionally, drinking enough water ensures that your digestive system functions properly by flushing out toxins and waste matter.

It's easy to mistake the sensation of thirst for hunger. So, if you feel worn down, tired, or sluggish, grab a bottle of water instead of a snack. Decide how much water you want to drink daily. A good rule of thumb is to aim for eight, eight-ounce glasses of water a day. If you sweat while exercising, drink a little more. You can also add fresh fruit such as lemon, lime, or strawberries to your water to switch up the flavors. Infusing flavor makes your water more interesting and helps you keep drinking.

Drinking Alcohol

Alcohol consumption has long been a popular activity, but it is important to understand the negative effects it can have on the body. During the COVID-19 pandemic starting in 2020, society at large began drinking more frequently due to stress, being home every day, and the convenience of same-day delivery service.[117] In addition, the lack of physical activity and increased snacking while at home all contributed to an increase in weight.[118]

A 2021 poll by the American Psychological Association found that 42% of US adults who responded, reported gaining more weight than intended since the start of the pandemic.[119] The average weight gain among this group was 29 pounds, with 10% reporting gaining more than 50 pounds during the pandemic.

Alcohol is a psychoactive substance found in beverages such as beer, wine, and spirits. It provides some energy when metabolized by the body, but is not necessary for good health and can be harmful when consumed excessively. As a toxin, it is important to use caution and understand the proper uses and limits of alcohol. The effects of alcohol on health can vary depending on the type consumed.

Moderate consumption of wine (up to one glass per day for women, and two for men) may reduce the risk of heart disease and certain cancers, but excessive consumption can increase the risk of liver damage, high blood pressure, and certain cancers.[120]

Moderate consumption of beer and craft beer may also reduce the risk of heart disease and type 2 diabetes, but excessive consumption can increase the risk of liver damage, high blood pressure, and certain cancers. Hard liquor, such as vodka, whiskey, and rum, generally have higher alcohol concentrations and carry greater health risks, including an increased risk of liver damage, high blood pressure, and certain cancers when consumed excessively.

It is important to remember that the potential health benefits of alcohol are only seen with moderate consumption, and excessive consumption can have serious negative impacts on health, including addiction.

Drinking alcohol can contribute to weight gain in several ways. While all types of alcohol can contribute to weight gain, beer, especially craft beer, can be particularly problematic due to its high calorie and carbohydrate content. A standard serving of beer (12 ounces) contains about 150 calories, while craft beer can contain anywhere from 150 to 300 calories per serving.

In comparison, a standard serving of wine (5 ounces) contains about 120 calories, and a serving of hard liquor (1.5 ounces) contains about 100 calories. It is important to be aware of the calorie and carbohydrate content of craft beer, and to consume it in moderation as part of a healthy lifestyle that includes balanced meals.

Other effects of alcohol include the decrease your testosterone levels. Moderate alcohol consumption (1-2 drinks per occasion) will not significantly decrease testosterone production. However, consuming more than 3 drinks in a single sitting can temporarily decrease testosterone by 6.5-20%. Testosterone is important for building lean muscle mass and reducing body fat. Repeated heavy alcohol consumption can lead to a range of health problems, including damage to the intestines, stomach lining, and liver, as well as problems with nutrient intake.[121]

Even if you choose to drink alcohol, you do not have to give up your favorite alcoholic beverages during your weight loss journey. Understanding how alcohol is metabolized can help you feel confident, and make informed decisions about your alcohol consumption.

Common Mistakes to Avoid in Your Weight Loss Journey

There are many common mistakes that people make when it comes to weight loss and maintaining a healthy lifestyle. Low calorie diets, not eating enough protein, only focusing on the scale, keto and low fat diets, snacking, not tracking foods, not having support, eating out too often, sleep and stress, meal planning, not drinking enough water, and alcohol consumption are all factors that can impact your weight loss journey. It's important to remember that there is no one-size-fits-all approach to weight loss, and finding a plan that works for you and your lifestyle is key. By avoiding these common mistakes and making small, sustainable changes to your daily habits, you can achieve your weight loss goals and improve your overall health and well-being.

Chapter 15

ℓℓℓ

Taking Action: Your Journey Starts Now

Congratulations on finishing *Beyond Feel Great*! You now have valuable knowledge and tools that can help you take control of your health journey and make positive changes. The purpose of this book is to provide guidance to those seeking answers on their health journey. My hope is that it will inspire readers to take action towards a healthier and happier life, viewing dietary mistakes and life challenges as opportunities for growth and progress.

The next step is to commit to yourself and set realistic goals for the future while keeping in mind that obstacles may arise. However, with determination and perseverance, you can overcome them. To inspire you to take action based on what you have learned, I want to leave you with a thought-provoking question: What will it take?

What resources, support, or changes in mindset and behavior do you need to implement the insights, strategies, and knowledge from this book into your daily life and fulfill your health goals and desires?

Asking yourself this question can help you recognize the challenges and opportunities ahead so that you can overcome them. Grab a pen and paper and be truthful and specific when listing the answers to this question and what is necessary for your success. Remember, it all starts with a question: What will it take? As you move forward, find a champion who can support and encourage you. Share this book with them to help them understand and support your goals.

Embrace change, even if it means facing pain and discomfort, as these sensations can motivate and inspire us to take action towards improving our health. When considering making lifestyle changes or reducing medication, it's essential to consult with your healthcare provider to ensure your safety and well-being. Discussing your goals and plans with them can help you create a safe and effective plan for change.

If your healthcare provider is interested in reading *Beyond Feel Great* and you would like to provide them with their own copy, please send an email request to doug@dougcollinsonline.com. Include both of your names, phone numbers, email addresses, and full mailing addresses; as well as your healthcare provider's area of specialty. Unfortunately, many healthcare providers do not view health and wellness in the same way as described in this book. However, if your healthcare provider is open to learning innovative new ways of approaching health, I look forward to sending them a copy of this book.

Stay committed to your health goals and use everything you've learned from the book to achieve optimal health and wellness. Thank you for joining me on this journey to go beyond just feeling great and live your best life.

Footnotes

Beyond Feel Great is a comprehensive guide packed with science-based information, designed to help you achieve your health goals. The book covers various aspects, from understanding body systems to nutritional advice and adopting healthy lifestyle tips. The author has painstakingly ensured that the content is both accurate and up-to-date. Throughout the book, you'll find extensive footnote references that support the shared health principles. For a complete list of references, visit beyondfeelgreatbook.com.

The author frequently cites products that have been pivotal in his personal health journey and daily routine, and which he recommends. It's essential to note that, to comply with government regulations and compliance policies, the book does not include specific product brands or company names. However, the author, being an authorized representative, earns affiliate commissions through the sale of these products, and he would appreciate your support should you decide to purchase any of them. If you're interested in learning more about these products to enhance and support your health journey, please visit the website beyondfeelgreatbook.com or contact the author directly via email at doug@dougcollinsonline.com.

About the Author

Doug Collins is a seasoned entrepreneur, author, and transformational coach with a career spanning over two decades. His entrepreneurial journey began in the late 1990s when he set up his own website to promote a line of wellness products and educational materials. Despite it being a part-time side project, Doug's venture quickly expanded into an international online business. In 2010, after a successful 22-year corporate career, Doug seized the opportunity to transition into self-employment, dedicating himself full-time to his home-based business.

With a persistent drive for continued knowledge and a keen interest in wellness, Doug has earned certifications as a nutrition consultant, metabolic health coach, and emotion code practitioner. As the author of *Beyond Feel Great*, he is passionate about inspiring others to achieve their goals and live life to the fullest. The transformative power of the information contained in his book is evidenced in Doug's personal journey toward improved health, demonstrating the possibilities that can be unlocked through focus and consistency.

If any health principle in *Beyond Feel Great* has positively impacted your life, Doug would love to hear your feedback and personal success stories. Similarly, if you have any suggestions on how he could improve the book, he values and encourages insightful feedback. To share your thoughts or ask any questions about the book, you can reach Doug via email at doug@dougcollinsonline.com or directly through the website beyondfeelgreat.com.

Made in the USA
Middletown, DE
01 December 2024